Thoughtful Dementia Care™:
Understanding the
Dementia Experience

by

Jennifer Ghent-Fuller

Thoughtful Dementia Care™: Understanding the Dementia Experience

By Jennifer Ghent-Fuller

ISBN – 13: 978-1480007574

ISBN – 10: 1480007579

Printed by Amazon CreateSpace.

This book is also available as an ebook.

website: http://www.understanding-dementia-experience.com

Acknowledgements

I gratefully acknowledge the support and encouragement of my husband, J. David Fuller, and my children, Sandra and Daniel. My sincere thanks to the six people who read and evaluated this book: Joanne Carruthers, Colleen Gildner, Stasia MacLeod, Doreen McMillan, Bernice Patterson and Lee Stones. Their feedback and words of encouragement were extremely valuable. I would also like to acknowledge Dr. Helen Creasey, whose video "The Brain and Behaviour," which was produced by the University of Sydney (Australia) Television Service for the Alzheimer's Disease and Related Disorders Society (ADARDS), started me on the journey of helping carers understand people with dementia. The support and encouragement of the many readers of my 2002 paper, "Understanding the Dementia Experience," who called and wrote to express their thanks, has been instrumental in my pursuit of a better way to explain the situations in which people with dementia and their carers find themselves. Finally, the people with dementia and their families, with whom I worked, were my greatest teachers.

This book is dedicated to people with dementia
and those who care for them.

Table of Contents

Introduction

Alzheimer's disease and other diseases causing dementia slowly steal all memories and abilities that have been learned since infancy - a process of progressive, permanent amnesia. All dementias are characterized by progressive brain failure due to brain cell deterioration and brain cell death. There is no cure for dementia at present. As the brain deteriorates, the person's ability, understanding and behaviour go through many changes.

Often people with a dementia such as that caused by Alzheimer's disease are seen as individuals with behaviour problems. It is important to reframe how people with dementia are viewed. When I first began to work in the area of care of people with dementia, I noticed that much of the reference material was about how to cope with the challenging behaviours of people with dementia. It was written from the viewpoint of the people looking after them. I set out to help myself and others understand instead, the viewpoint of the person with dementia.

If caring for people with dementia is challenging, how challenging is the experience of the people who have dementia? Firstly, they are people with an altered view of reality due to the Alzheimer's disease (or another disease causing dementia). Secondly, they are people, whose behaviour can change, depending on how we interact with them. In order to know how to interact with a person with dementia, it is important to understand what they are experiencing as a result of having dementia.

Once we understand the dementia experience, and no longer view people with dementia as having behaviour problems, we are able to see their behaviour as appropriate within the context of the dementia. This allows us to approach their care without fear. We can then deliver palliative care, care appropriate to someone with a fatal illness, with love and kindness.

For those readers who have dementia, or whose family members have dementia, this is emotionally difficult reading. Please remember that you have a lot of living left to do. You will need to find different ways to do things, but it is important to look for joy and hope every day. There is an enormous amount of research being done on dementia, with new research being published daily, and reason to hope for new treatments being available in the future. There is joy to be found in one's friends and family, in the beauty of nature, in the enjoyment of daily events, and in shared laughter. There is pride and contentment to be found in caring for a loved one, even though they have changed and become unable to do the things they did in the past. So please read to understand, and then turn your thoughts to the positive.

The initial draft of this document was written in 2002 to explain to family members the changes in the way people with dementia act and think.

For many years it has been distributed freely and also made available in 'pdf' format online as "Understanding the Dementia Experience." Since then it has received wide circulation and many people have written to say how much they appreciated the insight they gained through reading it. It also served as the outline for my family teaching sessions for many years. However, some topics that are important were not covered. In view of the need to think carefully about the experience of the person with dementia, and also to be thoughtful in terms of showing kindness, this new version is entitled Thoughtful Dementia Care™: Understanding the Dementia Experience.

One woman with dementia, who lived thousands of miles from me, read the 2002 paper online and sent me a very kind email. She was very thankful to have something to show to her husband and her sister that would tell them that she was not just being lazy or not trying hard enough, but that the way she was functioning was because she had been diagnosed with Alzheimer's disease. Another fellow, a relative to whom I was very close, said to me, "I hope I never become violent toward my wife." I replied that I would help her understand how to interact with him, so that this would never happen. His thanks were heart-felt. Many things in this book were difficult to write, but they were written in the determination to try to help make day-to-day life for the person with dementia and the carers, with whom they live, more understandable and, therefore, less stressful.

Originally, this material started out as a talk I wrote, which was based on the video "The Brain and Behaviour," featuring Dr. Helen Creasey, produced by the University of Sydney (Australia) Television Service for the Alzheimer's Disease and Related Disorders Society (ADARDS). The content has grown in depth and complexity (and hopefully insight) thanks to the people with dementia and their families who have discussed their experiences with me over the years.

The descriptions of memory changes I used in teaching and counselling were designed to be easily understood by family members. A formal survey of the academic literature will yield more precisely defined categories and differing views on how various memory processes and losses should be defined.

In this document, the emotional effects of dementia on the family have been woven into the discussion of the changes of the disease. Certain parts of this material evoked a strong emotional reaction from family members during teaching sessions in which I described the physical, emotional and psychological changes of people with Alzheimer's or other diseases causing dementia. At that point, we stopped and discussed their emotional responses. Therefore, the discussions of the emotional effects of this illness on the family have been deliberately placed with the emotional state of the family reader in mind in order to be wholistic and mindful of their reading experience. In fact, I often suggested to people that they read only as much of the original paper as they could handle. After that, they could delay reading more until they had spent some time thinking about it. After a few hours or days, they could go back to read more.

In order to be useful to everyone in the family and to people whose first language is not English, the use of complex medical terminology has been avoided or carefully defined.

The changes that take place in the person's abilities have been followed through to the end conclusion, in order to illustrate how everyday life changes as the disease progresses to the later stages. It is difficult to read about how your family member will be living at the end of the disease process. However, there were many people, who said, after talks or family sessions, that they wished they had had this information available to them years earlier. It is important to know what your needs, and the needs of the person with dementia, will be in the future. There are also some serious issues that can arise along the way. These are difficult to read about and consider, but much less stressful to cope with if you are aware of the possibilities.

Many family members have also told me that this knowledge helped them to stop feeling so frustrated in the early stage of the disease. Instead, they began to cherish all the abilities that their family member still had and to celebrate the family activities they were presently enjoying, rather than thinking only about what they had lost.

This text attempts to allow the reader to vicariously experience the phenomena of dementia, to step into the shoes of their family member with dementia - the confusion, anxiety, fears and realities of dementia - in order to deepen their logical and emotional insight and understanding. While the pattern of memory loss in Alzheimer's disease is the topic of discussion of the section concerning "Memory Processes" of this book, those who are dealing with memory loss due to other degenerative diseases, which cause memory loss, will also be able to recognize some aspects of this pattern and gain insight into their own situation.

A brief note on the terminology used in this book may be helpful. The term 'carer' is used in preference to the words 'care giver' and 'care partner.' This is done for brevity, but also to respect the fact that most family members do not start out thinking of themselves as 'care givers.' Rather, they are husbands, wives, sons, daughters and friends, and other people label them as care givers or care partners. However, if they are involved with the person with dementia, it is because they care.

Rather than use the words 'he' or 'she' or 'him' or 'her' or 'himself' or 'herself,' I have chosen to use the third person plural ('they,' 'them,' 'themselves') as the singular. I found out by reading in the Globe and Mail (a newspaper in Toronto, Canada) Stylebook that this was grammatically permitted, and find it preferable.

I worked for many years doing educational talks and supportive counselling. Someone in the audience at almost every talk I gave asked: "What is the difference between Alzheimer's disease and dementia?" Dementia refers to the destruction of brain cells and the pathways that join them as a result of a disease process. Common diseases that cause dementia are Alzheimer's disease, Lewy Body disease, Frontotemporal dementia, Vascular Dementia and Parkinson's disease with dementia. There are dozens of less common diseases that also cause dementia. The symptoms of dementia are related to the consequences of having areas of the brain that are no longer functioning. Consequently, there are many similarities in the symptoms of dementia, no matter which of the progressive degenerating diseases is causing the damage.

There are many stories of people with dementia and their family carers in this book. When I used such stories in talks, people always commented how much the stories helped them to understand the concept I was trying to explain. Whenever I asked families if I could share their stories anonymously, they were always very eager to make this type of contribution to helping others. I am very grateful for their generosity. Some details have been changed in the stories to ensure that they are anonymous.

1. Memory Processes

Most people think of their memory as one function and believe that they either have a good memory or a bad memory. However, there are many types of memory processes. The immediate, short-term, long-term, emotional and procedural memory processes are the main types discussed in this book. These different memory processes are organized in different areas of the brain. Some memory processes are affected early in Alzheimer's disease, and some stay intact for a long time. Whether a particular memory process is changed depends on the location of the brain damage caused by disease.

It is usual for the person with Alzheimer's disease to show changes in their short-term memory first, because that area of the brain is damaged first by the Alzheimer's disease. As the disease progresses, it affects more and more areas of the brain, and the family sees more changes in the person. Other diseases causing dementia also result in loss of the short-term memory, but it is usually not one of the first symptoms, as it is in dementia of the Alzheimer's type.

Some people have a rapid disease progression, and they pass away after only two or three years from the time their first symptoms appeared. Others have a slow progression, and live for ten to twenty years with the disease. As a general rule of thumb, if you notice changes every month, it is a very rapid progression. If the disease is progressing slowly, you may notice changes only every six months or so. You may not even notice the changes at all, because they happen so slowly, and you may only hear about them from family who don't see the person very often. People who have not visited for a few months or longer, are more likely to see a large change from their last visit, than the person who is experiencing very small changes from week to week.

Family members who are new to coping with dementia may expect that a person will be consistent: that when one type of memory is working well, the other types will also be working. We are used to all the memory processes coordinating our knowledge and memories so seamlessly that it seems like a single process. Our expectation is that a person who remembers what school they went to as a child will also remember how old they are now, what they had for breakfast this morning, and how to dress themselves, since they have been doing it for decades. So it presents a confusing picture when a person is able to have a good memory at times and at other times, it feels like they can't remember anything. Knowing the types of memory processes, the patterns of understanding they create, and the functions that are disrupted when these memory processes are not available, is vital to understanding the world of the person with dementia caused by Alzheimer's disease and other diseases.

1.A.Immediate Memory

Immediate memory is that which you use in conversation to remember what has been said just during the time period of the conversation. Think about any recent telephone conversation you had with a friend. If either of you had repeated yourselves, the other person would have remembered that the same sentences had already been spoken and wonder why you were repeating yourself.

Typically, people with Alzheimer's disease have an intact immediate memory during the early part of the disease process. They are able to use their immediate memory while the conversation is happening. Therefore, others usually find them coherent and socially acceptable. However, they may not remember later that the conversation took place or what was said, if their short-term memory is not good.

One fellow related a story about a fairly lengthy conversation he had with his wife. Prior to this conversation, he said how badly he was feeling that he had never told her that she had Alzheimer's disease, and wondered if it was too late to do so. I made the suggestion that he wait until she brought the issue of her poor memory into the conversation and then gently tell her. He did so, and they proceeded to have a long talk about what her diagnosis of Alzheimer's disease would mean to the family, including the possibility that she may eventually need to move into a long-term care home. She told him that if he could no longer look after her, she would want him to help her to make the move into a nursing home.

However, the next morning, when he referred to the Alzheimer's disease, she became very angry. She did not remember the conversation at all and denied that she had Alzheimer's disease or that he had ever told her about it. He was distressed, but after discussing the experience, he found some comfort in the knowledge that she had been able to let him know what her values and priorities were, even though she didn't remember telling him. This helped him when he eventually did have to place her in a long-term care home.

This lady had used her still-intact immediate memory to engage in a very meaningful conversation with her husband of many years, but her short-term memory loss prevented her from remembering that this pivotal conversation had ever taken place. This type of situation leads to a feeling of loneliness in the family member who still has intact memory. Companionship in a relationship involves being able to talk over the day-to-day events in the family and in the community. Family members who are emotionally close rely on each other to discuss the day-to-day changes and effects of tragic situations in the family. When one of the members of the conversation cannot remember a previous topic, further discussion of it will bring puzzlement, denial, hurt, and fear if they worry what might be

Thoughtful Dementia Care:
Understanding the Dementia Experience

happening to their memory. When one of the couple has dementia, the spouse, who is well, feels emotionally unsupported, as if they were alone. One fellow said, "She's still company, but it's just not the same."

Dementia is a tragic situation. Often spouses need to look outside their marriage, to other family and friends, for emotional support. Other people, whose family members are also experiencing dementia, are often extremely effective at supporting each other emotionally, provided they are in a professionally supervised group. Many people have said they don't know how they would have gotten through the experience without their monthly support group meetings.

People who do not live with the person with early Alzheimer's disease sometimes think that because they can have a good conversation with the person whose immediate memory is intact, there is really nothing wrong at all. When a question is asked of a person with dementia, such as "How are you?" they often answer with familiar phrases such as, "Fit as a fiddle, never been better!" They have retained the ability to know what answer will be well received, or socially appropriate, even though they forget what they are responding to very quickly.

A lady related a story of how her husband, who had been coping with Vascular Dementia for many years, and whose memory processes were severely affected, received a phone call from his brother. She was also in on the conversation on an extension phone and listened to her brother-in-law relate the happenings in his own life. Her husband responded very briefly with such comments as "Oh, yeah!" or "Oh, really," or "Is that right?" All of his responses were socially appropriate. After her husband had hung up, her brother-in-law said to her "See? There's nothing the matter with him! He understood everything I was saying!" This lady knew, however, that five minutes later, her husband would not even remember that his brother had called.

This misperception of the situation by family members who do not live with the person is very difficult for the one who is mainly responsible for their care, the carer. At the same time they are feeling a loss of companionship, they may also be faced with a lack of understanding and support from other family members.

Some family members will blame the deterioration of the person with dementia on the carer. They may say something like, "If you weren't doing so many things for Mom, she wouldn't be losing her independence." The carer has had multiple experiences showing that their family member can no longer perform certain functions. They know that if they don't take over and do some things, those things won't get done. They are being thoughtful, and yet at the same time, are being unfairly criticized.

The family members who are critical are basing their assessment on short telephone conversations during which the person with dementia has seemed normal because of their intact immediate memory. They may have had short visits during which the person with dementia is mainly listening and observing, but not interacting much and not actively trying to perform tasks. Many carers also related that in the very early period, the person with dementia could sometimes try very hard and perform very well, especially if they are in the presence of infrequent visitors or professionals. They find this exhausting, however, and cannot maintain this level of functioning. If the visitors have not witnessed the slow, day-by-day deterioration, they are startled when they eventually see a change in their relative. It is natural to resist acceptance of such deterioration, because it is emotionally painful to do so. The carer has no choice. They have to live with and deal with these changes.

At the same time, the carer is usually involved in visiting doctors, trying to find out what is wrong, to get a medical diagnosis and treatment. In order to help get a diagnosis, they are forced to tell how badly their relative is doing, and they feel guilt that they are somehow betraying the person whose memory and coping are poor. Many times I met family carers who were reeling from the emotional pain that the early days and months of dementia cause. I cautioned them to be careful what they say and to be understanding of other family members. Their slowness in acceptance is caused by grief. Otherwise, the family can slip into patterns of anger and accusation and be ripped apart irreparably. You will want and need your family later, so try to avoid doing permanent damage to the relationships.

A person with early dementia looks quite well, and usually acts normally for short times in social situations. Only people, who are with them for extended periods, see evidence of the enormous changes that are taking place. Eventually, the situation worsens and the distant family members have no choice but to acknowledge it. The earlier the whole family learns about dementia, spends time with the person, accepts the situation, and 'comes on board' offering support and help, the better. Sometimes I suggested that the carer gently encourage other family members to have the person with dementia visit on their own for a few days or a weekend. While it is possible to miss seeing the changes over a brief phone call or a visit of a few hours, the decreased abilities of a person with dementia usually become clearly visible in a two or three day visit.

Many years ago families frequently related stories about their physician also being unable or reluctant to accept that the changes being described were a possible indication of dementia. Family members often talked about the fact that the person with dementia was able to carry on a reasonable conversation with the physician during their short office visit, and this led to a dismissal of their concerns. Often we would discuss each of

Thoughtful Dementia Care:
Understanding the Dementia Experience

the early warning signs of Alzheimer's disease (see www.alzheimer.ca) and write down examples of the changes that were taking place. When presented with such detailed written information, physicians were able to see that there was cause for concern. At present, more people are being diagnosed with Alzheimer's disease, and other diseases causing dementia, at an earlier stage in their illness. Now, physicians generally have a greater familiarity with the characteristics of a person with very early stage dementia.

Physicians also realize that many conditions besides dementia can lead to temporary confusion and memory loss. As we age, our minds and bodies become frail. When this frailty exists, drug interactions, infections, metabolic or chemical imbalances, taking medication that is inappropriate for the elderly (google "Dr. Beers Criteria" for a list of these medications), and many other conditions in the body, can cause temporary confusion and memory loss, also known as delirium. Physicians know that considering the possibility of a temporary delirium, the cause of which can be treated and reversed, is necessary before a diagnosis of dementia can be approached.

1.B. Short-term Memory Loss and Its Impact

The short-term memory fails early in Alzheimer's disease. As previously mentioned, although the person may be able to use their immediate memory to have a reasonable conversation, because of the failure of their short-term memory, they may not remember the details of the conversation, or that the entire conversation took place, even just a few minutes later. However, the short-term memory is also involved in many more of our daily functions besides remembering conversations.

The short-term memory is the type of memory that you use to remember what has happened today, what else you are planning for the day and the next few days, and also what has happened in the last week or so. If you tried, you could probably think back for about a week, and remember everything you did, all the meals you ate, and the conversations you had on the phone or in person. That is the practical limit of short-term memories. You would not be able to remember this kind of detail if you were trying to remember back six months. To remember some things that happened months or years ago we use our long-term memory process.

Short-term memory is the memory process that allows you to do many things at once, or 'multitask.' For example, when you are cooking breakfast, you can remember how long the eggs have been boiling, when the frying bacon needs to be turned, when in the process to turn on the coffee maker and start the toast, and when you can fit in peeling the oranges. In contrast, a person with short-term memory deficit can concentrate on only one thing at a time, and if a second thing distracts them, the first may leave their consciousness completely. Trying to concentrate on many things at once, as we do if we are multitasking, becomes difficult, and then impossible, for people with short-term memory loss. Think about the process of making breakfast described above. The cook has to remember to check on each item of food being prepared. They also have to recall all the steps required to cook each item from start to finish. Not only that, but they also need to use their short-term memory to remember which of those steps they've already done and what comes next.

People with short-term memory loss due to dementia usually stop doing complex tasks like cooking very early in the disease process. These complex tasks are very common in the work world. If a person is still working when they start to develop dementia, they often lose their job because they can no longer function the way they need to in order to complete their work. Speaking from my own experience as a nurse on a hospital ward, I had to remember the names, diagnoses, room and bed number, and general health conditions of a dozen or more people; also, what medications they got and when, what care and treatments they needed to receive and how well those went, whether or not I'd recorded all this information, what I needed to ask physicians when they arrived on the ward; and, still be cooperative with the many interruptions that happened every hour. Most jobs have similar complexities. They require a reliable short-term memory.

Many hobbies also require the ability to multitask. One fellow I talked to remembered how content his wife used to be when she was knitting. He would often urge her to knit and she would refuse. In order to knit you have to remember where you last left your knitting, whether you are currently knitting the back, left front, right front or the left or right sleeve of a sweater, what the repeated pattern of stitches is, and what row you have just done and what comes next. Knitters need their short-term memories to finish their project successfully.

Many people with dementia find themselves making multiple mistakes when doing their hobbies. They become increasingly frustrated at their decreased skill and just quit their hobby or say they don't feel like doing it. Sometimes families are able to help the person with dementia continue a simplified version of their hobby. To do this they usually have to be present and coaching or working along with the person to finish the project.

One family related to me that their Mom had always baked the cake whenever they had family parties. When one cake turned out very badly, because she added some ingredients more than once and forgot others, they thought she should stop. I encouraged them, instead, to assign one family member each time to help her with the cake. This would allow her to keep her role and her sense of purpose and usefulness in the family for a longer time. It would also provide each family member with a constructive visiting opportunity in which the person with dementia feels safe doing a familiar task with a familiar person. Asking the person with dementia to teach you how to make the cake is often a more successful approach, rather than offering to help them with an activity in which they are used to thinking of themselves as an expert.

Another lady asked her husband to put her ingredients out in the order that they went into her baking. She was careful to put each ingredient away as soon as she used it so she wouldn't put it into the batter twice. Eventually she needed more supervision, but she did extend her ability to bake for quite some time. This lady had a lot of insight into her condition; not everyone retains this amount of insight.

Hobbies are very complex tasks with many steps and we all rely heavily on our short-term memories to do them. Most people stop doing their hobbies very early in the disease process, often before they have been diagnosed. The necessity to remember multiple complex steps is beyond the ability of someone with short-term memory loss. People with dementia often achieve more success when they do simpler one-step activities, such as raking leaves in the autumn. One lady related how pleased she was that her husband had this activity. He could see the pile of leaves as well as the leaves on the grass and could do the same motion repeatedly to get the leaves on the pile. When he finished, the wind had caused more leaves to fall. He would do this task over and over until his wife decided that he'd had enough and call him back to the house.

Sometimes people without dementia complain that they are often forgetful. They are worried that their forgetfulness means that they have dementia. Unlike a person with dementia, someone whose memory is functioning normally may be forgetful, but they will remember what they have temporarily forgotten as soon as they are reminded about it. For example, if you go shopping for a windshield wiper, you may get distracted and also buy other items that you need for your car or your home. You may even forget to buy the windshield wiper altogether. However, the first time you turn on the wipers again, you will likely remember that you went to the store and forgot to buy what you needed. A person with severe short-term memory loss will not remember that they had previously gone to the store for this item, or even that they needed it, even when they are reminded. If they go to the store with a list, they may not remember that they have the list with them. Typically, people with short-term memory loss come home without some of the items on their list, even if they do remember to look at it once or twice. The forgetfulness that results from dementia is not a mild annoyance; it has severe consequences to the person's ability to function. Short-term memory loss often results in the person with dementia buying the same item over and over again, because they have not made the memory of already buying it. Depending on the resources of the family and the cost of the item, this may result in financial hardship. Bills may be paid many times over, or not at all.

If you make yourself a cup of coffee and then forget to drink it, you will remember having done so as soon as you see the cold cup of coffee. A person with short-term memory loss may have the insight to know that they must have made the coffee, because it is there, but not remember doing it. They may, however, pretend to remember. On the other hand, if they have no insight as to the way the disease is affecting them, they may wonder who came into their house and made that cup of coffee when they weren't looking because they have no memory of doing it. Repeated similar instances may result in a mistaken conviction, or paranoia, that someone is invading their home.

One lady related a story illustrating the severity of her husband's short-term memory loss. She set a nice hot meal on the table and she and her husband sat down to eat. During the conversation, she asked her husband if he would weed the garden at the side of the house sometime soon. Leaving his hot meal on the table, her husband got up, went out the side door and

Thoughtful Dementia Care:
Understanding the Dementia Experience

started to weed the garden. When she went out to ask him to come in again, she discovered that, after he started to think about the garden, he had completely forgotten that he was in the middle of eating a meal. This is a good example of a person with short-term memory loss only being able to concentrate on one thing at a time. You can understand from this story why many carers eventually learn to curtail the spontaneity of their conversation, and instead evaluate the effect on their loved one of what they are going to say, before they say it.

In the early stages of the illness, short-term memory loss can create stress, frustration, tension, and a sense of longing for the way things were in the household. Learning to stay calm and pleasant despite the difficulties with short-term memory loss is important. Others may observe that the person still has most of their abilities, and feel that the situation is 'not too bad' yet. In fact, the early stage is the most difficult emotionally. It is also a time when the risk to the person with dementia is very high, because they are likely to make mistakes with severe consequences without other people being aware of their decreased ability. Understanding that this risk is present increases the anxiety of the carer.

Repetitive questioning, the same question being asked many times in a row, is the hallmark sign of short-term memory loss. Coping with repetitive questioning is difficult. It is best to answer the question each time as though it has not already been asked. Often the repeated questions centre on a topic about which the person is anxious. One fellow repeatedly asked when they would have breakfast, even though they had eaten. He typically did this every day until lunchtime. His wife found out by accident that if she didn't clean up the breakfast dishes, but left them soiled on the table for him to see until just before she made lunch, he was less likely to ask the question. Seeing the dirty dishes cued him to realize that they had already had breakfast. She was a very fastidious person, and really disliked leaving a mess, but found that the relief she had, in not having to answer his question repeatedly, made it worthwhile.

Another lady related how she coped with her mother's repetitive questioning. Her mother often asked her about her bank accounts. Her daughter would explain everything to her: how her rent was being paid, how much money she had, and in which bank, and so on. Five minutes later the same question would come again, and then again and again. Now, it is really a function of the long-term memory that this lady couldn't remember whether she had any money and where it was. Think of how anxious and insecure you would feel if you couldn't remember that information for yourself. Many people have noticed that repetitive questioning increases when the person with Alzheimer disease is emotionally upset or worried about a specific situation. This lady's short-term memory loss prevented her from remembering her daughter's explanation about her money, or even that she had been given an explanation. This pattern of misunderstanding is sometimes expressed as "You never tell me anything!" because that is how it is perceived by the person with short-term memory loss. After laying out the bank books and patiently repeating the information countless times, her daughter discovered one day, that her mother could be distracted by a discussion about dogs. Her mother had always been extremely fond of dogs, so she found any conversation about them emotionally captivating. They would tell each other stories about their own dogs, her daughter would tell her about friends' dogs or those she'd seen on the street. What the daughter found was that if she started to talk about dogs right after she had nicely finished the explanation about the money, it changed her mother's mood. Instead of being anxious, she was filled with pleasure and excitement. The money situation still had to be explained, but not nearly as often.

Using distraction in this way takes advantage of the fact that a person with short-term memory loss is only able to keep one thing on their mind at a time, and gives them something else to occupy their thoughts. Something with emotional appeal will be more effective, such as a soothing ritual of a cup of tea, or playing with the dog; whatever activity that is meaningful and pleasurable to them. Pull them gently into whatever activity you are doing to socialize. For example, you might say, "I would really appreciate your help chopping the vegetables," or "Would you mind handing me the nails while I fix this shelf?" Take them on an emotional journey by interviewing them about their early life. If you know their childhood stories, you will be able to say, "I remember you telling me..." and reminisce as if you were there yourself. Such conversations may bring back remote childhood memories that could be quite enjoyable for the person to talk about. Of course, if much of their childhood was emotionally painful, some other topic should be chosen.

I often suggested to families that they think of a few funny family stories, for example: "Remember the story that Aunt Minnie used to tell about sneaking into the house just before midnight, and turning back the grandfather clock to eleven o'clock, only to have it wake everyone up by striking twenty-three times?" Carers can use stories like this when the person with dementia is anxious and repeatedly asking the same question, or needs to be distracted because they are in a situation that makes them nervous. It is helpful to think of these stories ahead of time, as it is difficult to come up with a story when you are feeling frustrated and anxious yourself. You don't have to think of a different story for each time; the same stories can be used over and over again. Although this may seem manipulative, the person with dementia no longer has the ability to problem solve their way out of a difficult mood or pattern of behaviour. Changing the conversation to help them to get into a good mood and to be relaxed is like giving them a precious gift.

Why is it important to answer the repetitive question each time as though it has not been asked before? This is done to avoid humiliation. An example of this is the story of an elderly woman in a nursing home, who every morning, about half an hour after breakfast, would quietly say that she hadn't eaten that morning. She was offered a muffin and accepted that. In another half hour she would quietly say that she hadn't had any breakfast. She was offered a banana, which she accepted and ate. This was her daily pattern. One day when her daughter was visiting, a new care worker said to her "You've just eaten!" Quickly another staff member took the care worker aside and said, "We don't humiliate people in here," and explained this lady's breakfast ritual, and the thoughtfulness of her care.

Very often it is the tasks that are completed daily, like eating lunch, that people have the most difficulty trying to remember whether in fact that task has already been completed on that same day. The wife of one fellow insisted that he help her make the bed every day to help keep him active. Every morning, as they were making their bed together, he would scold her for having made it untidy again, thinking that they had already made it that same morning. Rather than argue with him, she would make up a reason that it was messy, such as having gone back to bed herself for a mid-morning nap.

People with dementia cannot remember that they have asked a question repeatedly, but they are quite capable of understanding that they are being criticized and scorned and are able to have feelings of sadness, humiliation and despair as a result. This is a very difficult disease to have, and it is important for the rest of us not to make the experience worse than it already is.

It can be helpful to people with short-term memory loss to put up white boards and use erasable markers to write reminders. Placing the board where it never needs to be moved helps the person with dementia find it, and they will go looking for the information they know they will find there (using procedural memory). One story illustrates this. The husband of a lady with dementia worked out of town in various locations on a daily basis. She had always found security in knowing where he was, even before she developed Alzheimer's disease. However, she would repeatedly ask him before work where he was going to be working that day, with barely a few seconds between the answers and repeating the question. At my suggestion he put up a white board on which he wrote, "Today I am working in _____" and he would put in the name of the town each day, for example, Cambridge.

On a later visit, he was asked how the whiteboard was working. He said it didn't work, because instead his wife would repeatedly look at the board and say "Oh, I see you're working in Cambridge today" with the same frequency with which she had previously asked the question.

Discouraged, he had stopped writing on the board. I asked him what his wife's response was to this. He thought about it and then responded, "She wrote it on the board herself." One could imagine that she visited that board quite frequently during the day, each time reassured that she knew where her husband was working. He and I were looking for two different results. He was hoping for the white board to improve her short-term memory. I was hoping for the use of the white board to improve her emotional security.

Another function of the short-term memory is to keep us oriented to the day of the week. Knowing what day it is usually constitutes one of our first thoughts after we awaken. Almost everyone has a strong habit of needing to know all day long what the day and date are. While it might take us a moment to figure that out, we usually remember what day it is for the rest of the day. People with short-term memory loss are not able to hang onto that information and often repeatedly ask during the day "What day is it today?" This is a valuable piece of information to put on a white board. Many families related how their family member with dementia would miss appointments or go to an appointment on the wrong day. People with dementia often appeared at the office on a day when their support group was not scheduled. It is useful to develop a method of providing them with a schedule at the beginning of every day.

Many families try to get the person with dementia to use a calendar, thinking that if they cross off the day before, they can keep themselves oriented. However, this is something a person with short-term memory loss cannot do. They cannot remember if it was today or yesterday that they crossed off the previous day. In order to use a calendar, one needs to remember what yesterday was. Calendars can be successfully used only if someone else crosses off the day before and the person with dementia gets used to (with their procedural memory) always being able to rely on the first date that is not crossed off. Even then, a calendar is often cluttered with too much information, which causes a person with short-term memory loss to become confused about what is important and what can be ignored. Some people with short-term memory loss I have known have developed a habit of looking at today's morning paper for today's day and date, and they check it repeatedly during the day. Others have found a channel on the television which always has the day, date and time showing twenty-four hours a day. Not everyone has the abilities remaining to take such steps, but they can be very helpful for months or years for those who do.

Taking medications is difficult when a person has short-term memory loss. They may remember taking pills, but not that the last time was yesterday, or many days ago. So they may miss many doses. Or they may not remember taking a pill and take it more than once. Was it yesterday or today that they took their pill and ticked it off on the calendar? What day is it today, anyway? Having the person with short-term memory loss fill up their own pill organizer or dossette is not always a reliable system, although many family members reported that their loved one continued with great determination and care to do this for themselves for as long as possible. The time comes, however, when despite their best efforts, they are unable to be accurate and need someone else to take over one more step in the process. One lady refilled the dossette as soon as she had taken her pills, so it became impossible for her family to check that she was taking them properly. Many people described a complete disorganization of the medications when the person with dementia was responsible for them: pills mixed up in each other's containers, evening and morning pills in the wrong area of the dossette, or pills all over the table or counter. Because these medication mix-ups happen early in the course of the disease process, it can be difficult to persuade the person with dementia to give up this area of responsibility. They are still quite capable of arguing and trying to find ways of doing without the offered help, and they may not realize that they are making errors.

The first 'level' of medication supervision is usually counting the pills that are left and asking the pharmacist to be notified if the prescription is being refilled too often or too seldom. Once there is evidence that the person with dementia is being inaccurate with their pills, the family often change their care by putting the pills in the dossette themselves and keeping the pill bottle unavailable. As the effects of dementia intensify, family members have to change their care to actually giving the person their pills each time. There are tamper-proof automatic pill dispensers available for purchase, which have voice announcements that it is time to take a pill, and systems that can allow a family member to view on-line whether the person has taken their pills (for example www.carelinkadvantage.ca). Medication supervision is one of the highest priorities for care resulting from the short-term memory loss. Since this loss is often present as an initial symptom, the taking of medications is an early safety issue. Taking multiple doses, or not taking their medications can result in severe illness or death for the person with dementia.

In the beginning of the disease process, the short-term memory sometimes works and sometimes doesn't. This can be frustrating as the person and their family cannot rely on consistent remembering or consistent forgetfulness. Family often assume that the person will not remember, and this may offend the person with dementia, whether or not they do remember accurately at that particular time. As the disease progresses, people with dementia completely lose their short-term memory. I often compared this inability to hang onto memories to pouring water through a sieve. The information just doesn't stay. It is very important to understand that this is due to physical changes in the brain and not due to laziness or lack of trying.

A state of high anxiety will decrease the ability of the person with dementia to use their remaining immediate and short-term memory skills temporarily, and they will return to their new normal after they are calm. Family members who had been constantly criticizing or arguing with the person with dementia, but then learned how to interact in more positive ways, often noticed that their loved one with dementia was much more relaxed once the number of arguments in the household decreased, and their anxiety diminished.

We also use our short-term memory in order to learn new things. We hold the new information in our short-term memory, and each time we practise or review the memory, it becomes stronger. Finally, the memory becomes permanent and part of our long-term memory. A person with a short-term memory loss is often unable to learn about new things or new procedures. One family bought a microwave for their mother when she kept burning things on the stove because she would forget that she was cooking. They thought that she was being stubborn in not using the microwave and in not trying to remember how to use it. In reality, she had lost the capacity to remember the instructions, no matter how many times they were given. Someone who had already been using a microwave for many years would be more successful in using it instead of the stove. Burning things on the stove is quite common in people with short-term memory loss, because they start to do something else and forget that they are cooking. If they go for a walk or lie down for a nap, a fire can result. Many family members take the fuse out of the stove if the person with dementia will be home alone. They also help the person with dementia to practise the procedure of knowing to leave if the smoke alarm sounds. This is another serious safety issue in the early stage of dementia, if short-term memory loss is involved, and one that is not easily fixed.

One fellow lost his job many years ago when his company required the staff to switch from using calculators and account books to using computers. No matter how much training he had, he could not learn how to use a computer. He was diagnosed with dementia of the Alzheimer's type two years after he was forced into early retirement.

Another family got a new television and showed their mother, who had Alzheimer's disease, how to use the remote control. Each time she wanted to watch a show, she would hand them the remote control and tell them which show she wanted to see. This family became increasingly quite annoyed, eventually yelling at her that they had already told her how to use the remote control. When the effects of short-term memory loss were explained to them, they were very remorseful at their treatment of their mother and felt a huge amount of guilt.

Many families feel remorse and guilt for their treatment of the person with dementia. Four things about learning how to care for someone with dementia are important to realize. Firstly, most family carers are unfamiliar with the effects of dementia on people's abilities, and people with dementia due to Alzheimer's disease, or another disease, function in ways that most of us have never experienced. Common sense does not help here. The carers have to learn how to understand new information about memory processes and how to cope with situations that are new to them.

Secondly, don't be too hard on yourself. If you realize you have made a mistake in the way you have been interacting with a person with dementia, learn from it, change what you are doing, but don't hang onto the guilt. Forgive yourself. Know that every family goes through these painful experiences and feelings of being inadequate. Apologize to the person with dementia and then distract them with something fun.

Thirdly, understand that each person with dementia is unique in the way they behave and how they understand what is happening. What has helped one family carer to cope may not help the next. Be patient with yourself and the person with dementia and never stop trying to find ways to help yourselves. Coping often means trying one thing after the other, and then using the approach that works for as long as it continues to work.

Fourthly, scolding and arguing will not help them learn because they have lost most of their capacity to learn with their short-term memory. Scolding will, however, establish a procedural memory in their mind that interacting with you is always unpleasant.

Dementia due to Alzheimer's disease or another disease is a progressive illness. When an approach or a care pattern, that has been successful, stops being effective, it is usually because the person's abilities have changed due to deterioration in the form of further damage to the brain from the disease. Carers become aware of the change when something goes seriously wrong. Calm yourself down, and then try to figure out what step in the procedure the person with dementia can no longer do. This will help you go through the process of finding a new approach that you both find acceptable. For example, for many months, a son may have left meals in his father's fridge for the coming week. One day he comes with meals for the next week and finds that his father has eaten only two from the previous week. He may try phoning to remind his Dad to eat. He may ask his Dad to heat something in the microwave and then observe his ability to do that. He may need to change to clear containers if he finds his Dad no longer realizes that the packages in the fridge contain food. Thinking about all the skills that are needed to do the task, and then evaluating the person's ability to perform each one, will help to figure out which step is no longer available to them.

It is important to realize that, no matter what your approach, the person with dementia will not regain the skills and knowledge that they have lost and will need to have more and more things done for them. Caring for someone with dementia involves creating the conditions that facilitate the person with dementia doing as much as they can for themselves, and knowing which things they absolutely need done for them. It is emotionally difficult for the carer, because they work harder and harder, and the condition of the person with dementia continues to worsen.

For example, one lady noticed that her husband was no longer reliable in remembering to shave, comb his hair, brush his teeth and wash his face in the morning. He still knew how to do each of those tasks, but was forgetting to do them. Putting a checklist on the mirror helped him for many months. He could see in the bathroom mirror whether his hair had been combed, for example, and was able to use the list to check whether he had done everything, despite his short-term memory loss. They worked this plan out together, and because of her gentle approach, he did not mind this list being put on the mirror.

Eventually, as the disease progressed, he was no longer able to do these tasks for himself, but having the list allowed him to keep more of his independence for longer than he would have done otherwise. Keeping one's independence for as long as possible, helps a person maintain their dignity and their sense of usefulness. While it might seem easier to just do it yourself, the person with dementia may become more irritable if they do not have useful activities that they can do independently or with help. This may lead to frustration and irritability, especially if they resent receiving help they feel they do not need.

Part of the stress of coping with dementia is dealing with constant change, a relentless diminishing in the person's abilities and understanding. There is what I call 'a fine dance' in helping people who are losing their ability to do tasks. They are not doing it properly; can you decide it is not doing anyone harm and praise them for a job well done? They need help, but do not want to accept it. Can you figure out a way to approach them to help without causing them to feel insulted or useless? Maybe it involves discussion; sometimes it is better if no words are spoken, but the assistance is offered in a nonchalant, relaxed way. I knew one proud couple who were in their nineties. They were retired hard-working farmers. He became very upset if his wife urged him to have a bath and helped him wash. He saw this as being treated like a child. She altered her approach, instead saying "it's time for our bath," and climbed into the tub with him. This was successful until he was no longer able to climb in and out of the tub, and she needed to find a new way to help him stay clean.

The family whose mother needed them to operate the remote control for her became very angry. Grief and anger are closely related. The carers who are frustrated by how often they lose their temper, often discover that they are feeling a huge amount of grief concerning the changes in their

Thoughtful Dementia Care:
Understanding the Dementia Experience

family member. Once they are able to identify that it is grief that they are feeling, they are often able to help themselves by allowing themselves to feel and express their sadness, and this decreases their tension and helps them to avoid angry yelling.

I often found that as family members listened to me tell about the changes that take place with dementia, asked questions and made comments, they would suddenly burst into tears. They became suddenly overwhelmed with the devastation that the disease was causing in their family member. Many people came to learn about dementia because they did not like the fact that they were angry, and speaking crossly, and wanted to change their approach. Learning about the full course of this devastating disease often allows the family to realize that they are feeling grief. This sadness gives family carers a sense of appreciation for the abilities their family member still has left, and what activities they can do together, rather than looking back at what is missing or being irritated by the mistakes the person with dementia is making. Family carers are also then able to develop a sense of pride in how they are able to help the person with dementia.

Loss of the short-term memory also causes a change in thinking patterns in the person with dementia. If you consciously focus on what you are thinking at any time during the day, you will likely find that you were thinking about what had already happened that day, what you still have to accomplish, who you need to talk to, or what has just happened or is about to happen in your life. All of this information is stored in your short-term memory. It is not very often that we think about our remote past unless something reminds us of it. Since daily events are no longer stored in the minds of people with short-term memory loss, they spend a lot of time thinking about the memories that are still available to them. Usually, this is about the past. Consequently, much of their conversation is also about the past.

Family members who are experiencing the effects of dementia for the first time are sometimes frustrated because they cannot have discussions that develop over days, weeks or months. Examples would be how a child is doing in school, how an expectant mother is coping with her pregnancy, or how a political candidate is faring during an election campaign. Each new piece of information builds on all the previous knowledge you have about the situation, and you are able to evaluate how you think things will turn out. It becomes impossible to try to have this type of discussion with a person who doesn't remember what grade the grandchild is in, whether their daughter is pregnant or that an election is coming up. You have to re-establish all the information to have the conversation within the bounds of their immediate memory. The next time you want to talk about it, you need to do it again. Sometimes it feels worth the effort, sometimes not. The need to talk about ongoing concerns is a legitimate need of the carer. If they are no longer able to meet this need with the person with dementia, it may become important to them to find another person to have these types of conversations with, in order to meet their own needs.

The person with dementia also has a need for social conversation. However, family members often become upset because the only thing the person with dementia wants to talk about is the past. Actually, it's often the only thing they are able to talk about. However, once family and friends accept this, and learn that conversations about past events can usually be successful, they find that there is a lot to discuss. A person with dementia may spontaneously and repeatedly tell the same story about their past. When other long-term memories besides that one are spoken about, family members often discover that the person with dementia has a lot of other memories that can be triggered by specific questions, comments, or the reminiscence of others. When you do this you are helping the person with short-term memory loss feel joy and contentment instead of emotional pain, and you will enjoy your day considerably more as well. It helps them replace their worrying thoughts with pleasant and engaging thoughts. People without dementia can do this for themselves, but people with short-term memory loss due to dementia need someone to help them get away from constant worrying.

At one family dinner table, everyone but the person with dementia would chat about current events. The person with dementia wouldn't really pay attention, because the conversation had no meaning to him. He would occasionally interrupt and start talking about something he had suddenly remembered. It might have been an event that happened over forty years ago. Initially, he was scolded for interrupting the person who was speaking, and for trying to force a change in the topic of conversation. Once they learned about the changes in memory processes, the family changed their approach. They would, instead, talk about the topic he had brought up until that conversation was finished. They had intact short-term memories. They could pick up their former conversation at the exact point where it had been interrupted. Their family member with dementia was pleased and satisfied that he had contributed to the conversation and had a successful social interaction experience, which he needed. The family were pleased to provide this for him.

The person with dementia cannot adapt their behaviour, because this requires intact brain processes. The person with dementia will not learn to avoid interrupting and await their turn to talk. They are not mindful of the conversation around them because it has little or no meaning to them. They may have developed a procedural memory that, if they don't say what they are thinking immediately, they will forget what they were going to say. However, they may also develop the habit of not talking at all because they get scolded each time. We are the ones who need to change our behaviour to adapt to the changes in the person with dementia.

Interruption by the person with dementia is a useful procedure for families. This is a thoughtful way to include the person with dementia. If they wait politely until another person finishes speaking, their short-term memory loss will prevent them from participating in the conversation. "Just interrupt us whenever you want to say something" is the procedure. Establishing procedural memories is discussed in the section entitled "Procedural Memory." After they have made their comment, it is often possible to finish your discussion and then turn to the person with dementia and say, "Now, you wanted to talk about _____." You are functioning as their short-term memory.

Since the short-term memory is affected early, many people who are developing Alzheimer's disease are misunderstood. In dementia of the Alzheimer's type, long-term memories are preserved in the early stage. Often they cannot remember what took place five minutes ago, but they can remember what took place sixty, seventy or eighty years ago, sometimes with great detail. For this reason, family and friends may suspect that the forgetful person really does know about recent events too, but is pretending not to remember. They may say to themselves, "If he can remember what happened when he was five, why can't he remember what we talked about ten minutes ago?" They expect consistency between memory processes because our memory processes are normally consistent and integrated with each other, until we develop Alzheimer's disease or another disease causing dementia. Until one understands that different memory processes and pathways are involved, the memory problems of dementia can be very puzzling.

Short-term memory loss results in emotional upheaval for the person with dementia. If someone calls to say they are coming over, they forget and they are surprised later when that person comes to the door. Most things that happen to them are unexpected because the person with dementia does not remember that they are going to occur. This constant experience of having the unexpected happen becomes a procedural memory of "Nobody ever tells me what is going to happen next." This can lead to severe anxiety and distress. The anxiety and distress are more likely to occur if other people react with anger or impatience, showing their surprise to the person with dementia, by saying something like, "What do you mean you don't remember, I told you yesterday!" Learning to control your reactions is very difficult and takes a lot of time, patience and creativity.

One family member taught herself how to crochet to avoid becoming angry. If her mother had an appointment, she would arrive over an hour earlier than usual to take her there. While she reminded her mother repeatedly where they were going, and that she needed to continue to dress herself to go out, she worked on her crocheting to prevent her frustration from building.

It is difficult to avoid making the person with dementia feel as though they are being 'bossed around.' Staying pleasant and calm, introducing humour, singing together, distracting them with conversation about other more interesting issues as you coach or help them with their bathing or dressing, can be very helpful, both to the person with dementia and to yourself.

I have often talked to family members about the futility of arguing with a person with short-term memory loss. We all argue at times with people who are close to us. Think about an argument or discussion where you had a difference of opinion with someone recently. You both state your opinion and then you go back and forth, restating and qualifying what you think. Hopefully you resolve your differences. However, both of you need an intact short-term memory to know what the discussion was about and what each of you said. Without an intact short-term memory, a person ends up after the discussion with the viewpoint that they started with, and will forget that a different conclusion was reached.

Gently introducing new ideas in a repetitive way, which takes advantage of remaining procedural memory skills, is one method of coping with this issue. At other times, trying to avoid the topic altogether seems like the only option. For example, quite a few families ended up in arguments about the car formerly owned by the person with dementia. Having lost their driver's licence, they were no longer able to drive and had given or sold their car to a family member. However, when they later forgot this transfer of the car's ownership because of their short-term memory loss, they then accused the person of having stolen the car. Families quickly figured out that the person who now owned the car should not park it in their grandparent's or parent's driveway, for fear of starting the same argument again. This type of event often shocks families. It is important to realize that it is normal for a person with short-term memory loss to make this kind of error. Their surprise and accusation is no different than yours would be if someone took your car without permission. They have no memory of giving their permission, so as far as they are concerned, they didn't.

Being thoughtful about dementia care means keeping in mind what will disturb a person with dementia. One daughter related that her Dad would walk to and from the adult day program he attended. He had always done a lot of walking around their town, and was quite reliable at that point in time to get himself there and home again. She noticed that he would invariably be in a very happy mood when he got home, but wondered why within about five minutes, he would be grumpy and hard to get along with. I asked her if she could remember what their typical conversation was after he got home. She said, "Not much. I just ask him what he did that morning." When she asked him this, he realized he could not remember what he had done that morning. This would frighten him and cause him to feel a sense of failure, hence putting him into a bad mood.

If the person with dementia has severe short-term memory loss, a new carer, or any visitor, coming into the home may find it necessary to reintroduce themselves several times during each visit. I recall visiting one couple in which the woman with dementia and short-term memory loss could no longer speak, but she could understand most of what was being said. She continuously wandered around the house and every time she entered the living room where her husband and I were conversing, she would be startled, and concern and displeasure would cloud her face as she looked at me. Each time this happened, I would get up, walk over to her with a big smile and warmly shake her hand while I introduced myself and stated why I was there. She would then walk about the living room for a short time, smiling, and then leave for other parts of the house. This pattern was repeated several times over the course of my two-hour educational visit. Short-term memory loss makes it very difficult for people with dementia to adapt to changes. Carers who work in the home have said that it takes many frequent and regular visits, progressing slowly and in a very friendly manner, until the person with dementia gradually builds up a procedural memory and accepts their presence.

Misplacing items is another consequence of short-term memory loss that is very annoying for people with dementia. Their short-term memory loss prevents them from recalling where they put something. When they need it the next time, they are unable to locate it. This happens many times a day and is very frustrating for the person with short-term memory loss and their carers. One fellow, who had developed short-term memory loss during his Vascular Dementia, designed a solution for himself that worked for a couple of years. He took a red placemat and placed it on the hall table. On this placemat he kept his wallet, keys, glasses, false teeth and comb. He tried very hard to always put them there and succeeded most of the time. This eliminated many hours of searching for lost items every day.

Thoughtfulness means noticing the effect on the person with dementia when you say or do something. If you notice a negative reaction, think carefully about what has happened, put it into the context of your knowledge about dementia, and try something different the next time. If you get a great reaction to something you said or did, remember what it was so you can do it again, and share your insight with the rest of the family. For example, one fellow found that taking his mother out to feed the birds always helped her become calm and happy. He could not get his own tasks done when she was agitated. If he continued to try to do his personal tasks anyway, both of them experienced increasing frustrations and the build-up of negative emotions. He got more done in the long run if he took the time to help her become calm.

Unfortunately, some family members feel that it is alright to tease the person with dementia and to make fun of their memory loss. This can cause the person with dementia to feel angry and irritable much of the time. The constant irritation and frustration that the person with dementia feels in this circumstance makes it difficult for them to continue to use their remaining abilities and to cooperate with their carer as they go through their day.

Some activities do not require use of short-term memory but can be enjoyed 'in the moment,' without remembering what has just happened or what is about to happen. Reading short poems, or writing them together, is one example. Watching sports is often successful. The score is often at the bottom of the screen and the fast-paced action can be captivating moment by moment. Recorded sports shows in which the commercials and intermission have been removed would hold the interest of the person with short-term memory loss longer. Many people with a short-term memory loss like to watch the same show over and over, and a recorded show has the advantage of always being available when it is wanted, rather than having to say "there's nothing on television right now." Also, other ways to occupy the time such as going for a walk, watching a fire in the fireplace, being outside in nature, and playing with a pet, are examples of activities that we all enjoy and that do not require us to use our short-term memory.

People with dementia and short-term memory loss may have great difficulty keeping themselves occupied or entertained, and this is a huge issue for carers. Reading a book, for example, loses its meaning because the person with dementia cannot remember what happened in previous pages or chapters. People with short-term memory loss become bored when watching a television drama or a movie when they can't remember the plot, the characters, or the previous events. They lose interest and wander off, or start talking. Since they are not able to enjoy the show, they lose sight of the fact that others are concentrating and enjoying it. If they are asked not to talk, they will quickly forget and start talking again. Being unable to entertain and occupy themselves, they look to those around them to provide activities that will help them feel accomplishment and usefulness. This is wearing on the carer. For this reason, having the person with dementia spend time with other family members or attend a day program becomes a necessity for the well-being of the carer.

It has been mentioned that the change in thinking due to short-term memory loss includes the tendency to become distracted very easily and the lack of ability to keep more than one thing in mind at a time. There are other elements that increase the effects of these changes.

The brains of those with Alzheimer's dementia become very slow in processing information. If you are waiting for a person with dementia to respond to you, you may notice that they take an unusually long time to do so. Typically, we are used to rapid responses and we become uncomfortable when there are silent pauses in a conversation. At this point, we often fill the silence by adding additional information or qualifying what we have said. If we add additional information while waiting for a person with dementia to respond, we are going to distract them and make it harder for them to respond. It is better to learn to become comfortable with the silences.

The brains of those with dementia also eventually lose the capacity to sort relevant from irrelevant information. If you go into a store, for example, you may be intent on finding a new shirt. You will focus on finding the right store, then the shirt section, and then finding the colour and style of shirt that you want. You are ignoring the other items in the store, the other people, the music and other noises in order to focus on your task. A person with dementia, who cannot identify what information their brain needs to concentrate on, in order to find the shirt they want, will quickly lose their focus on the task.

So the effect of the short-term memory loss and the distraction it causes is compounded by the slowness of processing information and the inability to sort and ignore irrelevant information. Some people with dementia who are in a store or plaza, or another situation where there are many things to be seen, heard and touched, drift from one thing to another and seem aimless. Keeping track of their location is necessary, since they may forget where they are and who is with them. Others become overwhelmed and agitated by the situation and may demand to leave. When this happens, there is no option but to take them home and, if it happens consistently, to make arrangements to leave them at home when you shop. In the early stage of the illness they may be fine on their own, especially if you write on a white board where you are and when you'll be back. Later, if they can no longer be left alone, you will need to find someone to keep company with the person with dementia while you shop or work.

If a person with dementia becomes overwhelmed by too much happening at a family event, they will want to leave and it will cause conflict for the carer who wants to stay and visit. Many families cope by setting the person with dementia up in a quiet room and taking turns by having one person at a time go in to visit with them. This accomplishes the necessity of the carer to keep their social contacts and interaction, as well as the need for the person with dementia to avoid situations that are overwhelming.

Going to a restaurant can be very challenging for a person experiencing these changes due to dementia. Pretend you are a fellow with early memory loss going out to lunch with his daughter. Think about how you approach a menu. There may be between two and eight pages of possible meals you can order. You are supposed to decide on the category (hot meal, sandwich, salad) of food you are going to eat, and that narrows down your choice. If you have decided on a salad, for example, then you have to choose which salad you prefer. If you approach this task with a short-term memory loss, you may forget what was on the previous page each time you turn to the next page. You are not able to go through the process of slowly narrowing down your choices to a specific item, because you can't remember what the possibilities are. Maybe you try throwing out a suggestion, such as "I'll have a hamburger." only to be told in a hushed voice, "Dad, this is a vegetarian restaurant!" Then you ask your daughter, "What are you having?" thinking that might help you decide. "Artichoke soup," you are told. You hate artichoke soup. "But I don't like that!" you reply. The response comes back "Why does it matter whether you like what I am ordering for myself? Pick something that YOU want!" But you find the menu confusing and you are overwhelmed. Not only that, but there are a lot of strangers in this room, moving about and talking loudly, and that is making it even harder for you to concentrate. You are wondering whether you know the fellow across the room and you forget that you are trying to pick what you want for lunch. Then the waitress comes and says, "What would you like, sir?" You have no idea, so you say to your daughter, "What are you having?"

So many families described this type of difficulty in a restaurant that I began to ask regularly if it was happening. Many times they were puzzled when the person with dementia did not remember the context in which they were situated. They may have been sitting in a familiar restaurant that serves only seafood, and everyone felt uncomfortable when the person with dementia ordered steak. Many family members found ways to cope. They learned to decrease the confusion by making sure they were in a quiet corner with the person with dementia facing the least active area, such as the window, so it was easy for them to concentrate on only the people at their table. They gave subtle suggestions, such as, "You really enjoyed the fish and chips the last time we were here, would you like to try it again?" One lady found that this worked for a couple of years, but then the activity was so confusing for her husband that he became agitated. Eating out to have a change of scenery was very important to her. She then began to pack picnics, and they took them to a quiet park instead of struggling with the environment of the restaurant.

The loss in their abilities means that the person with dementia has a very tough time getting through their day. They are trying to remember, processing slowly, reacting to getting things wrong and to other people being upset. They are not sure what to do next and want to figure their day out. This is very difficult, if not impossible to do and the person with dementia has to concentrate as hard as possible to do their best. For this reason, they are often seen as self-centred. In my view, trying to also keep track of another person's needs and limitations is yet another thing to be remembered and taken into account by their short-term memory. Because of their short-term memory loss they are able to think about only one thing at a time; doing one thing and simultaneously thinking about how it is affecting someone else is multitasking: trying to do two things at once. It seems beyond the ability of most people with dementia to be thoughtful and considerate of others when they have so many other things they cannot remember to do for themselves. This self-centredness is not intentional on the part of the person with dementia. It happens as a result of their loss in mental abilities.

Being thoughtful about the person with short-term memory loss means helping them compensate for that loss in the events of their daily life and being mindful of the emotional changes that accompany this loss. Carers need to approach the person with dementia in a way that helps them to relax, to feel safe and secure. Helping them to stay safe in the use of medications and use of the stove are a high priority. Being gracious, when the person with dementia is forgetful, means: answering a repeated question as if it was the first time of asking; refraining from reasoning and arguing; and, neither expecting them to remember, nor becoming upset when they forget.

1.C. Long-term Memory Loss and Its Impact

To remember back many months, years or decades, we use our long-term memory. An intact short-term memory is sometimes used to make new long-term memories. We can also make new long-term memories with our procedural and emotional memory processes and this will be discussed later. Using our short-term memory process, we revisit and rehearse the daily events in our lives. If something is insignificant to us, happens only once, and we never think about it again, we usually don't remember it over the long term. However, if we rehearse and repeat a new piece of information, or think frequently about an event that has taken place using our short-term memory processes, the memory or the ability becomes a strong, permanent, long-term memory. We learn it.

After the short-term memory is affected by dementia, the individual with Alzheimer's disease does not usually make many new long-term memories about events that have occurred. Short-term memory loss interferes with being able to learn new information because each time the person is presented with the information, it is as though it is the first time they have seen it. The process of revisiting and rehearsing that information cannot start because the information is not retained.

At the beginning of Alzheimer's disease, the individual has a fairly intact long-term memory, but they are not adding many new memories to it. However the long-term memory is also slowly erased. The typical pattern of this in Alzheimer's disease is that the most recent memories disappear first.

If a seventy-five-year-old has had Alzheimer's disease for two years, they may have vague memories of their life between age sixty and seventy-five, but clearer recall of their first sixty years of life. As their disease progresses, they may have access only to the memories of their first fifty years, then their first forty, then their first thirty years, and so on, until they can only access their childhood memories.

This is not an orderly reversal – the person may remember more or less on different days, and at different times during the day. Sometimes their minds skip about from decade to decade, and even combine parts of memories from one stage of their life with another.

The slow erasure of long-term memories backwards in time, also referred to as retrograde amnesia, results eventually, in the person with Alzheimer's disease sometimes thinking they are much younger. It is not as though they realize they are, for example, eighty-one, but they can only remember their first thirty years. Instead, they expect to be in the same context that they were at age thirty. Consequently, they are confused, because they may not recognize their family, since they are looking for the individuals they were sharing their life with at age thirty. They may also be looking for the same home they lived in earlier, or expect to go to work at the same place at which they worked forty or fifty years earlier.

The long-term memory loss of the individual with Alzheimer's disease leads to the family coping with many unique and unusual situations. One lady forgot that a family feud existed. She and her sister had an argument, decades earlier, and the two families had not spoken to each other since then. Her sister was quite surprised when she started calling and visiting frequently. Fortunately for all concerned, her sister decided to go with the flow of the situation and re-established relations so she could be part of the family circle caring for this lady with Alzheimer's.

Another family talked about the months their father spent sitting and crying. His past experience of living as a prisoner in a death camp controlled by fascists was all he could think about and talk about for that period of time. They could distract him temporarily, but he reverted to thinking about that painful period in his life over and over again. The family saw it as a blessing when his disease progressed so he was no longer consumed by such difficult memories.

Another lady seemed to see the residents in her nursing home unit as her children. She was able to walk and would take them down the halls in their wheelchairs saying, "We have to hide, he's coming!" Her grandchild related that this lady had been unable to protect her small children and herself from a physically abusive husband. Calming her meant making her feel that both she and her children were safe from her husband, who had actually died many years before. Many people, who have lived through abuse, the terrors of war, torture, and other emotionally and physically painful situations, experience enormous anxiety and terror when their mind tells them they are back in that context. Sometimes we have no way of knowing what that background may be, even with a family member. It is important to be soothing, and to somehow make them feel protected, rather than trying to argue about what is real. The fear is real to them, and they have a need to be validated and to feel safe.

A woman described to me the despair she had felt, thinking that her husband was troubled and miserable since he could not remember so much of his past. One day she visited him in the nursing home and asked him what he had been doing that day. He replied he had been riding his bike with his brother. He smiled when he said this and talked about what a sunny day it was and how much he had enjoyed riding his bike beside the sea. She had peace of mind after that, knowing that he was dwelling on the pleasant thoughts of his childhood in another country.

One might compare our reality to a jigsaw puzzle. We have all the pieces in place, and we are able to see the whole picture. The longer a person has Alzheimer's disease, the more pieces are missing, and the more difficulty they have in understanding the picture.

However, it is human nature to try. A person with dementia may look at their thirty-year-old daughter, and decide that she must be their sister. They only remember their sister as she was at age thirty, not as she is now at age fifty or sixty. They may remember their daughter as she was at five, but not recognize her as she is now at thirty. Therefore they may call their daughter by her aunt's name. Misidentifying family members happens with almost everyone with dementia due to Alzheimer's disease.

Not being recognized is hurtful and grievous for family members. However, realizing that the person with Alzheimer's disease is desperately trying to put them into context may bring some understanding and emotional comfort. It is typical for a person with Alzheimer's to forget the youngest members of the family first, as they are the latest additions to the family, and the most recently made memories are erased first. They may remember them, but not their names and whose children they are. They may say "What lively children! Whose children are they?" If you answer, "THEY'RE YOUR GRANDCHILDREN!" sounding upset or angry, you are likely to cause them to feel humiliation and frustration. This may lead to them becoming antisocial, since socializing becomes unsafe in their procedural memory. They will form a new habit of not talking to the people around them.

It is vital that the grandchildren be told that not being recognized does not mean their grandparent does not love them. Neither should they push their grandparent to try to remember their name as this will be frustrating and increase their sense of failure. It is better to use everyone's name in the conversation as much as possible, as the person with dementia may still be able to quietly orient themselves about who they are with, given that subtle assistance.

As the person with Alzheimer's disease continues to be increasingly relegated to the context of their own past by the advancing of the disease process, they eventually experience the present as if it were their own childhood. One woman thought that the retirement home she was living in was her childhood home. She was very distressed at all the strangers who had invaded her home and convinced that they were the ones who had taken away all the furniture she remembered.

It is extremely common for people with Alzheimer's disease to be looking for their parents, and to be very distressed if they are told that they are long dead. They no longer have access to the memory of the event of their parents' deaths and funerals. Thinking of the context of the person with Alzheimer's disease, it is as though one is telling a ten-year-old, which may be the age they think they are, that their parents are suddenly dead.

They become sad and upset. Then, because of their short-term memory difficulty, they ask again for their parents, being unable to remember that this conversation took place a few minutes ago. If they are again told that their parents are dead, their anxiety and sadness is increased. What does a child do when they are upset? They look for their parents to comfort them.

The more upset the person with Alzheimer's gets, the more they need the reassurance they hope their parents will provide. They may become angry, because they 'know' perfectly well that their parents are not dead. Living without all of their long-term memories changes what is true or real about their past in their minds. They develop a different version of reality, a different context to their lives, than the rest of the family has.

If another person continues to insist that the parents are dead, the person with Alzheimer's disease may experience an escalation of their frustrations and emotionality to the point that they may lose their temper completely and 'explode' in what has been termed a 'catastrophic reaction' (see the section entitled "Catastrophic Reactions"). This is best avoided, as it is emotionally painful for the person with the disease and their carers. One lady became extremely upset when she was taken to her parents' graves in an attempt to convince her that they were really dead. She accused her husband and sister of conspiring to lie to her and she was inconsolable. She was so upset that she left the house when her husband wasn't looking. Quite by accident, she was spotted walking down a street by a family member who just happened to be driving by. This was a very painful episode for all the family.

A daughter was frustrated because her father repeatedly took everything out of the closet in his bedroom. The bed was placed in the room so that the closet was to the left of the head of the bed. She would put everything back into the closet and close the door in hopes that he would leave it there. She asked him many times not to take things out of the closet. As we talked about long-term memory loss changing the time context for the person with dementia, she suddenly remembered that when he was a child, his parents had to walk through the room where he slept to get to their bedroom. The door to their bedroom was in the same position, to the left at the head of his childhood bed, where his closet door was presently located. His daughter then realized that he wasn't creating difficulties on purpose by emptying a closet. In his reality, he was trying to go into his parent's bedroom to find them. For the next period of time, she left the closet empty to decrease her own stress. She was also able to understand that he needed reassurance and distraction when he was looking in the closet.

No amount of convincing and arguing will allow a person with dementia to grasp and accept another person's reality. An understanding of the changes in memory and psychological processes is basic to understanding the altered reality of people with dementia and in helping them to avoid emotionally painful situations. One lady with Alzheimer's dementia was told, whenever she talked about her parents, that they were in Florida. She missed them, but she was glad they were having fun in a nice, warm place. She still had the memory, which she made as a young adult, that her parents go to Florida yearly to visit family members, which made this story plausible to her.

Another family tells their mother that her husband has gone fishing every time she asks for him. He died many years ago, and she no longer remembers that he is gone. However, she does remember that he fishes almost every day in the creek behind the farmhouse where they lived when the children were young, and that he stays away for hours. So when she receives the information that he is fishing, she is reassured, her anxiety does not build up, and she develops the habit of feeling secure because every time she asks the same question, she gets the same answer.

Being aware of the reality, in which the person thinks they are, is important to looking after them. Some people are still able to verbalize how the world seems to them. One fellow with Alzheimer's, while visiting with his wife in his nursing home unit, commented to her "It's really hard being fourteen years old and in this prison with all these old people." Since hearing that statement, I have often wished that technological advances would someday permit caring for people with advanced dementia without resorting to housing them in locked units. Another time, he looked at their wedding picture, which was beside his bed, where he and his wife were sitting. Not recognizing that he was actually sitting beside his wife, he nodded at the picture and said sadly, "I'll never make love to her again." Most people do not retain their insight to this extent, but we can learn important lessons from those who do. We need to assume that even those who are not able to express such sentiments may also be experiencing them. Many researchers have written about the value of the validation of the experience and beliefs of the person with dementia, whether or not it is in agreement with generally accepted reality. This means to accept the version of events that the person with Alzheimer's has and to talk to them as though what they say is absolutely true. This is very controversial. There are many people who feel that telling a person with dementia something that is not true is lying, and should never happen. Others believe that it is important to give emotional support within the context of the reality that the person with dementia is experiencing, even if it means that they are not telling the truth. This is something that each family has to evaluate for themselves, and for the individual for whom they are caring.

Although it seems awkward at first, I have known many people who continue to live with the person with dementia for years, without that person remembering who they are. One woman's husband consistently called her Gramma, and thought she was his grandmother, but they were able to visit and do things together, nevertheless. A husband eventually labelled himself as a friend who was helping out. His wife would point at a picture of him taken fifty years before and say, "That's my husband! You're not my husband!" Another woman called herself, "the lady that your wife asked to look after you." She calmly explained this every time her husband asked for his wife, and then went on to other activities and topics. He often commented how surprising it was that she and his wife had the same first name. Now and then, he would insist on getting a message to his wife, and he was satisfied by talking to his brother or one of his children and asking them to get a message to her that he was alright. His wife left their numbers beside the phone for him and they were helpful in calming him down whenever he called. He had Lewy Body disease and early in the disease process lost the ability to identify his wife specifically, while retaining the ability to identify other family members.

These people initially tried to convince their spouse who they were, but later got used to being misidentified. Of course, they never stopped grieving the loss of not being identified. I found their dedication very moving. One fellow, whose wife was in long-term care, had some staff members discourage him from visiting. They said there was no point, because she didn't remember who he was. His reply was profound: "She may not remember who I am, but I remember who she is."

Even though a person cannot identify their family members does not mean that they have lost the need for the loving and caring relationship. One lady, whose husband had had Alzheimer's for many years, told me that she thought her husband had no idea who she was, and that her visits had no meaning for him. However, her daughters told her that his eyes followed her wherever she was. This told all of them that she was important to him, even though he couldn't express it. Many people described such behaviour. It indicates that there is more than one level of knowing a person. Whether or not they can state the person's name and say what their relationship is, they may still have the knowledge that they belong with that person and that they have a bond.

It is very difficult for family members when they no longer share the same memories as their loved one. I remember one woman looking at me very sadly when her husband told me proudly and happily that they had been married for seven years. In fact, they had been married for fifty-three years. I was present when a mother failed to recognize her daughter for the first time. She had only one daughter, who was sitting beside her as we chatted. She asked me if I knew when her daughter would be visiting her. Her daughter was absolutely stunned by this development.

Another lady felt very discouraged. She said that the more than fifty years she had spent happily married seemed to her as lost, as a complete waste of time, since her husband couldn't remember them. I pointed out to her that she would not have felt that way if he had suddenly died of a heart attack, and she agreed. Dying slowly of dementia often means that the grief the family members feel is prolonged, being added bit by bit as the person with dementia loses each memory and ability. Instead of losing him completely, she had to get used to having him present, when his memories were not present. Pauline Boss, author of a book entitled "Ambiguous Loss," and another book entitled "Loving a Person with Alzheimer's Disease," describes this pattern of grieving very eloquently.

Many people with Alzheimer's disease describe a heightened ability to remember their very early years. This happens for some people in the early part of the illness. One fellow said he could remember conversations with his mother and father word for word, which had taken place when he was six or seven years old. (When I asked if this was upsetting, he said, "No, it's kind of a nice visit!"). A lady was shocked when she suddenly remembered clearly the day her sister came home from the hospital as a newborn. She was only eighteen months older than her sister. Some people surprise their elderly brothers and sisters with the extent of their recall of their early family life. The explanation for this phenomenon in some people is unknown, but it is quite common to hear it described. Without access to the short-term memories to think about during the day, the thoughts that are available to think about concern the past. Constantly thinking about the past may mean that those memories become more readily available. Of course, this memory pattern leads to other people not believing that the person has dementia. They say things like: "If she can remember what happened when she was five, why can't she remember what happened five minutes ago!" Developing an understanding that there are many different memory processes and that one may be intact while another process is not, helps clear this misunderstanding.

Another thing that can be misunderstood is the habit many people with Alzheimer's disease have of covering up for their lack of memory. A fellow may spend an evening with good friends, laugh and chat and seem very appropriate, and then afterward ask his wife on the way home "Who were those nice people?" How could the person with Alzheimer's disease be so dishonest as to spend a whole evening with people and pretend to know them? From an early age, we are all taught to 'cover,' or hide, our memory lapses by pretending to know, until we do remember, in order to remain socially graceful. If you meet someone on the street, and you remember their face, but not their name, you will usually chat with them until you do access the memory of their name, and not let them know that you ever forgot. If you can get away with it, you will move into talking in vague general terms in order to cover up your memory lapse. You do this because in our society, it is considered rude to forget something important like a person's name, or significant events that happened to them. So we hide our forgetfulness to avoid hurting the feelings of others. People with dementia have not lost this long-ingrained habit; they just need to use it much more often than they ever have before. People with memory loss are not able to control when they forget something, and they may remember it one day and forget the same thing the next day.

The long-term memories that are affected by Alzheimer's disease are not only those for events, but physical memories or automatic abilities as well. As we progress through childhood and adulthood we learn about doing many things that become so habitual that we do them without consciously thinking through each step. Using cutlery, brushing our teeth, washing, toileting skills, grooming, dressing, driving, playing the piano, typing, skiing, skating, riding a bicycle, or swimming are all examples of over-learned or habitual activities that we may have practised so frequently that we do them easily without conscious thought. Since these skills are over-learned, they are usually maintained in the early stages of Alzheimer's disease, or another disease causing dementia. However, they will gradually be lost.

In our early life, we also learn what things are, and how they are used. If you look around the room you are sitting in now, you can name each object of furniture, you know how to use it, move it, and care for it. You can name the window, as a window, and know what you will see if you look out. People with dementia develop a total or partial loss of the ability to recognize familiar objects or persons through their senses as the result of physical brain damage due to the disease they have. Any of the senses can be affected. People with dementia develop an inability to identify something by sight, such as things that are in every home. People with normal hearing become unable to identify the sounds that they used to know well, such as a dog barking. They have difficulty using the information they know: they may be able to describe the furniture in a room, but have difficulty going around it as they find their way across the room. Even though they have been able to read all their lives, the words may look like mysterious squiggles on a page.

I find it useful to compare our long-term memory to a filing cabinet. As we go through life, we add information to the files, we put them in categories, and we cross-reference them so we can use the same information in different circumstances. The disappearance of the long-term memory is like taking file after file out of the cabinet and tossing it out. Below, are some examples.

One fellow was very early in his Alzheimer's disease, had passed the driving test required for eighty-year-old people, and his wife was still comfortable in the passenger seat when he was driving. He remembered the way to their destination, but his wife asked, "Aren't you going to turn left here?" He replied, "Yes I am." "Why haven't you put on your left hand turn signal?" she asked. "I just can't remember how to put on the signal," he replied.

He knew he had to signal his turn, but the knowledge of making the automatic movement of his hand, which he would have used to put the signal light on, was no longer available to him. That tells us that the brain cells and pathways where that memory is stored are being damaged. He may remember that skill occasionally over the next few days and weeks, if those cells are still partially functioning. However, when those cells are gone, he will never regain the memory. He will not be able to relearn it because his lost short-term memory process will no longer support this type of learning.

A lady with dementia recounted going to the mall with her husband. He walked into the mall, assuming that she was right behind him. He held the door open, only to find that she was nowhere around him. When he went back to the car looking for her, she was in a panic. She had suddenly lost the memory of how to open a car door. This experience had a big emotional impact for her. She needed a lot of reassurance that she would be looked after, no matter how badly she was affected by the disease. It sounds like a small thing, but it was a major crisis for her.

Since skills can be used only if all the memories needed are present, the loss of one small skill can mean a whole element of living has stopped. The fellow who could not remember how to put on a turn signal no longer felt confident that he could drive, and asked his wife to do all the driving from then on. He knew that she could help him with the turn signal, but he was afraid that the next thing he forgot when he was driving would be more significant, such as forgetting how to put on the brake.

Another fellow used to be able to cook well, but had lost the ability to do anything but make the tea. One day, his wife went out to the kitchen because he was taking so long. She found him puttering about, the water had boiled, but the teapot was jammed absolutely full of tea bags. He had gotten stuck and hadn't stopped putting tea bags in the pot. This is called perseverating. He also didn't remember that he only needed two bags.

If a person looks out the window and sees snow on the ground, they will automatically put on warm clothes when they go outside. However, a person with dementia may no longer be able to form the connections between the snow indicating it is cold outside, that they will feel cold if they go outside, and that they need warm clothing. Similarly, they may be perspiring on a hot day, but no longer remember that if they remove the heavy sweater they are wearing, they will feel cooler. The ability to understand their problem and figure out a solution would require that they are able to remember the significance of each fact and how the facts relate to each other in a situation.

I remember watching a small child become able to use the phone. She went from not knowing what the phone was used for, to thinking that the person who was speaking was actually, magically in the receiver. Finally, she realized that she could somehow communicate, by using the telephone, without the person she was speaking to being present. Step by step she was adding information about the telephone to her own 'filing cabinet' of long-term memories. The person with Alzheimer's disease or a related dementia goes through a similar process, but in reverse. Initially, they forget how to look up a new phone number, and only dial numbers that they know well. Later, they will answer the phone, but not make calls themselves. They will often forget to say when someone has called, so having the service of being able to look back to see who has called is very helpful at this stage. Eventually, they will refuse to use the phone altogether. Other inabilities such as lack of sound recognition, visual recognition, and language processing add to their memory loss until they reach the point where the person with dementia cannot use a telephone, something they have done for decades.

Mirrors are particularly troublesome for people with long-term memory loss who have forgotten what mirrors are and that you see your own reflection in them. Furthermore, if their memory context is back in time, they may expect to look twenty, thirty, or forty years old, and may not recognize themselves in the mirror at their actual age of seventy, eighty, or ninety. Mirrors are often placed in the hallways, the bedrooms and the bathrooms of a home, and often in the living rooms and dining rooms as well. The experience of a person with dementia who has lost the ability of interpreting the information provided by mirrors as they walk through their house must be like seeing a stranger pop into view and then disappear again every time they walk past a mirror and see their reflection, or the reflections of other people in the house.

Many family members talked about the person with Alzheimer's complaining that there were one or more strangers in the house or that people were breaking into the house. Sometimes their own reflection resembled that of an older relative that they didn't like, or they thought it was a stranger, and they frequently yelled at the image in the mirror to "Get out!" Covering the mirrors, with cloths or curtains, or just taking the mirrors down, often removed a major source of irritation, and brought peace back into the household.

Imagine an elderly man who goes into the washroom in his nursing home and comes out complaining about the other man who won't leave. The carer goes in with him and finds the washroom otherwise empty. He insists that the other man leave before he does his business. The carer is frustrated, because she cannot make this man understand that there is no one but himself in the washroom. This occurs many times a day, and the man's frustration slowly builds over the days to the point that he 'needs' sedation. Of course, this man no longer knows what a mirror is and what it does. Furthermore, his memory has gone backward in time, and he thinks of himself as looking the way he looked in his teens. So, each and every time he goes into the washroom, he sees an eighty-year-old stranger who refuses to leave as long as he is in there, and therefore he has no privacy. Even if the carer tells him that he is in the mirror, it will not help, as he has forgotten what the word mirror means, and forgotten the concept of reflections in mirrors, and forgotten what his face looks like in the present. Once the cause of the problem is figured out, the mirror can be covered, and the man will regain his sense of privacy and his frustration and anxiety will decrease. He needs others to work within his reality to help him solve the problem.

Some days, people with dementia will remember very little, other days it seems as though they are 'back to normal.' One fellow described his experience as feeling like there was a veil dropping down before his eyes, enveloping him in the darkness of confusion. When he felt clear-headed, he would ask his wife how long he had been 'gone.' He commented that at some point, he was certain that he would no longer return from this state of mental darkness. This phenomenon of seeming well again usually happens only in the first year or two after symptoms of the disease begin. When this happens, it often brings a strong grief reaction from family members as they get a glimpse of what they have lost.

People with dementia have good days and bad days. At some times, they will seem to be in the present, at other times back thirty years, at other times, back seventy years. It is very challenging for others around them to continuously adapt to the time frame that the person is forced to be in, by the disease. However, the ability to do so creates a supportive emotional environment.

One fellow I met was continually afraid of being arrested. Fifty years earlier, he had gone A.W.O.L. (Absent Without Leave) after being conscripted into an aggressing army. He did not believe in what the army was trying to accomplish, so he left. However, he could not remember that he no longer lived in that country, nor that the army into which he was conscripted, had been defeated decades before. There was no point in telling him this; the only thing that helped him was to reassure him that he was safe from being arrested. He did not start by telling his story. He repeatedly asked to have the door closed, and also wanted to know if anyone was looking for him. His eyes and his body language showed that he was in great fear. Viewing him, as merely a person who was paranoid because of his dementia, and dismissing his fears, would have left him trapped in his nightmare. Getting his trust to the point where he would share the cause of his fears permitted very specific reassurance that allowed him to relax. This would have to be repeated each time he started to worry, but without his carers having that knowledge, he would not have had periods of relaxation. It is important to listen to the themes and the emotional content in the conversations of people with dementia, in order to discover more information about what is causing them anxiety or fear.

Thoughtfully walking in the shoes of the person with dementia, with the changes in their cognitive processes in mind, will often lead you to discover what the source of their difficulty is, even though they are not able to clearly tell you. Watch their behaviour, and try to see how they are interpreting the environment in which they live. This is especially important if they are acting as though they are feeling threatened, and are trying to defend themselves.

Quite a few families related that the person with dementia had quit smoking years before. Suddenly, they went out and bought a pack of cigarettes. They began smoking again as though they had never quit. They no longer had access to their memory of quitting. The person with dementia often smoked more cigarettes during a day than they ever had before, since they forgot how long it had been since their last cigarette, due to their short-term memory loss. It is difficult to help the person with dementia to stop smoking again as long as they are able to go to the store independently to purchase the cigarettes. Carers had an easier time after the person became unable to shop. The person with dementia will often think about having a cigarette whenever they see the package or the used ashtray. The person with dementia rarely thought of smoking if the carer kept the package of cigarettes in the cupboard with the cleaned ashtray.

Some 'memories' that the person has may have actually happened to someone else, or came from a book or a television show, and instead, they recall these things as something they did. These 'memories' are termed 'false memories.' When this happens, it truly stuns the family with disbelief as they are sharply reminded of the enormous changes that are taking place as a result of the dementia.

For example, one lady, a widow who developed Alzheimer's disease, started talking to her family and friends about her past hobby of playing golf. This was very disturbing to her children as it had been their father who was the golf player, and their mother had never picked up a golf club. She had a huge store of memories of golf tournaments, but did not remember that it was her husband who had played in them.

When people who have some false memories tell untrue stories about people in the family to other family members, it is emotionally painful. If the others in the family believe those stories, then it can result in arguments, resentment, and anger. It is important for all members of the family to be aware of the possibility of this happening and to work together to get to the truth if the person with dementia is giving disturbing information about individuals.

The person with dementia is not always conscious of the erasure of their long-term memory, and therefore it does not usually bother them, depending on the degree of insight they retain. What is upsetting to them is that other people react with criticism, correction and disapproval. Being thoughtful means realizing that they have no control of how their memories are retained and going with the flow of their conversation by accepting it. One lady with dementia asked me whether she had ever been married or had children. I was startled by the question, but managed to smile and reply with the truth, that she had been happily married for over fifty years and had raised six children, who were all successful in their lives and visited her frequently. "How wonderful!" she replied, and went down the hall with a big smile on her face. If she had instead been criticized for not remembering such basic information, she would have been very upset.

People with dementia trust their memory. Your conversation will go smoothly if you give people the freedom to talk about their past as they remember it, rather than argue with them about what really happened. This is especially difficult for spouses to do, since most of us with spouses end up having these types of discussions throughout married life, without any dementia being present. The two members of a married couple seem to remember things differently because different aspects of a situation have more emotional impact on one person than another. We tend to remember those things that affect us emotionally, and if the event does not impact our spouse in the same way, we remember it differently. Therefore, learning to go along with false memories for the sake of the peace and security of the person with dementia often means 'unlearning' the habit of trying to get each other to agree on how past events happened, a habit which has been present for the entire length of the marriage. It means giving up the need to be right, which is very difficult for all of us.

Many people have wondered whether they should tell people with dementia when someone else in the family passes away. In my view, whether or not they will remember being told this, they have a right to know and should be told at least once. Regardless of the dementia, they still have full 'personhood.' It is not necessary to keep telling them over and over again to try to get them to remember it. Rather, if they mention it again, give the news in a matter of fact manner, but be ready with another story, or an activity to start right away in order to distract them. Whether you start saying something like "he's gone fishing," depends on how upset they are when you give the bad news again, and how obsessed they are with asking. You will have to use your own judgement and values to make that decision. It is important to come to this decision as a family, so that everyone is consistent. What can happen if a person with dementia is not told that a family member died, is that the other people in the family are very worried that they will 'let something slip,' by accidentally referring to the person as dead, and they become quite nervous when they visit. Eventually, this has led to family members ceasing their visits or coming by very rarely. This results in the person with dementia being abandoned when they are in a long dying process, when they most need their family around them, looking out for them in order to advocate for their well-being. Most families I met knew instinctively whether or not a person with dementia could manage attending the funeral of a family member or friend. By the time someone is elderly, they have gone to dozens of funerals in their lifetimes, so it is not an unusual event for them. If it is the funeral of someone they have been close to, it may help them if another family member speaks on their behalf, saying those things that they would have said, had they been able to do so.

The patterns of memory loss in other types of dementia differ from those in Alzheimer's disease. People with Vascular Dementia may maintain their short-term memory, or have it unreliable: occasionally working well and other times not working, until the middle stage of their disease or later. Their long-term memory does not show the chronological regression of Alzheimer's, instead there are gaps of years or topics that they can't remember. These people may remember much of their adulthood, but nothing of their childhood. Since Vascular Dementia is caused by multiple small strokes, the memories that are lost depend on where the strokes have destroyed brain cells, rather than rolling backward in time, like the Alzheimer pattern of long-term memory loss.

People with Lewy Body disease and Parkinson's disease with dementia also have memory loss, but since their disease process does not typically start in the area of the brain housing the short-term memory, the pattern of memory loss differs from those with Alzheimer's disease. People with Frontal Lobe Dementia have an intact memory until the dementia becomes more global, affecting a large part of the brain. In the early stage, they will remember being told not to do something, for example, but the area of their brain that enables them to make good judgements has been affected, and they will do it anyway and say they don't see why they should stop. An excellent and easy to read book on Frontotemporal Dementia is "The Banana Lady" by Andrew Kertesz.

Many people have more than one type of disease causing dementia. In these individuals, the pattern of memory loss is mixed. No matter what the pattern is, each individual has a unique understanding of the reality in which they are living. Their reality, in that moment, must be understood in order to help them feel cherished and safe.

Having many different areas of the brain affected results in a constellation of inabilities. Often people refer to a person's pattern of behaviour as resembling the rotation of a kaleidoscope. (I first heard this comparison from Marge Dempsey, of the Alzheimer Society of Niagara, Ontario, Canada). The development of one small deterioration can change the whole pattern of abilities that remain, and alter the behaviours of the person, as a result of the changes in their understanding of the world around them.

Regardless of which disease causes the memory loss, the effect of that memory loss on the individual's ability to understand where they are, whom they are with, and when it is in time, will be similar. The changes in ability, in understanding, and in behaviour are due to the resulting destruction of the brain cells by the diseases causing dementia, not as a direct effect of the disease itself. For example, whether the area of the brain that is responsible for short-term memory is destroyed by Alzheimer's disease or by Frontotemporal dementia, the individuals affected will have similar misunderstandings due to their short-term memory loss. The same kinds of changes happen with different diseases, but the pattern of when those changes occur differs from the general pattern of individuals with Alzheimer's disease. However, each pattern is unique to each individual with dementia.

1.D. Emotional Memory

Those events in which the person with Alzheimer's disease is emotionally invested may be remembered more easily. Events that have a high emotional impact do not need to be repeated and rehearsed in order for us to remember them. If you think back to many of your own long-term memories, most of what you recall easily, will have had high emotional meaning for you at the time it happened.

Think about what you remember from studying for a high school history exam. At the time you studied for the exam, if you reviewed the facts many times, you were probably successful in the exam. While you wouldn't do as well if you took the same exam today, much of what you studied will seem vaguely familiar if you read something about it or visit a historical site you studied. This is typical of a long-term memory established by repetition in the short-term memory process many years earlier.

Contrast that type of memory with the memory of where you were and what you were doing when the first manned spaceship was launched, when President Kennedy was assassinated, or when the World Trade Centre was attacked on September 11, 2001, or when a child of yours was born. When they recall such events, most people can immediately remember the room they were in, who they were with, whether they were standing or sitting and what they were doing at the time. Events that you remember most clearly from your past will likely be those about which you are very emotional. For example, many women can recall an enormous amount of detail of the day their children were born, even decades later. One of my own family members was very emotional about the cars he owned. He remembered the exact years in which the events of his life had taken place by relating them to what car he had owned at the time and how many years he had been driving it. In contrast to many other long-term memories, these emotionally laden memories are very clear in detail and depth.

For example, if you are learning a new phone number, you need to practise it in your short-term memory before you can easily recall it without looking it up. However, if someone tells you that a new baby is expected in the family, you learn this instantly. You do not have to practise and rehearse. This is the character of a long-term memory established by emotional mediation.

People with dementia, especially those in the early stages, even though they are usually not able to form new long-term memories because of their short-term memory loss, occasionally do so because the strong emotional impact alone is sufficient to make this new long-term memory. This phenomenon is known as emotionally mediated memory. For example, many people with dementia do not forget having their driver's licence taken away. Happy emotional times, like the job promotion of a son, or the birth of a grandchild, also often have enough emotional impact to be remembered, at least for a time.

Family members are startled by the ability of the person with dementia to remember one event when they are usually unable to remember anything at all that has happened in their daily lives. Normally, with no disease present, our memory processes are consistent with each other and support each other. When a disease causing dementia is present, it is surprising, after so much is forgotten, that one event is remembered. Often this incident is so meaningful to the person with dementia that they will talk about it over and over again. Some people use these exceptions, the few instances of a person with dementia laying down new, emotionally mediated memories, as evidence to claim that there is no disease process. They may say to themselves "If she can remember the kind of car we just bought, that proves that her memory is still working and she has no disease. She is pretending to be so forgetful just to be difficult." It is important to look at the whole picture, and the long-term patterns of the person's memory processes, rather than a few specific instances.

Here is an example of the emotions helping a person with middle stage Alzheimer's disease establish a new long-term memory. A fellow told of reluctantly leaving his wife behind, in the care of others, and making their annual trip 'home' by driving to the east coast alone. His wife had been diagnosed with Alzheimer's disease for about six years, she did not always recognize him, and she spoke very little. She felt very insecure travelling in the car and usually insisted on returning home after approximately half an hour. She was disappointed that she wasn't going on the trip, but he hoped that her faulty memory would protect her from some of the sadness at missing the trip. When he returned, he thought that his wife had forgotten that he had left her behind. However, the first time he cooked fish, she said, "You went home without me!" The smell of cooking fish triggered memories of the east coast trip she had missed. The memory came back only when she could smell fish cooking. This led to such a strong negative emotional reaction in her that he eventually had to stop cooking fish altogether.

Sometimes families hope to establish a new memory because it is emotional. However, there is no guarantee of being able to do this. One lady told a story about taking her father to his great grandson's birthday party. She was hoping that he would remember the event and his great grandson. What he remembered the next day was only that he had received a bag of candy from someone the day before. From her father's point of view, the outing had been a success and he had a happy memory as a result.

One lady with dementia due to Alzheimer's disease forgot to close the lid on the washing machine when she was doing her laundry, and her

Thoughtful Dementia Care:
Understanding the Dementia Experience

clothes did not get washed. This formed an emotional memory for her. She convinced herself that if she tried to use the washing machine again, she would break it. Her family tried their best to explain what had happened, but she could not remember their explanations because of her short-term memory loss. What she retained was a strong emotional memory that she had tried to do a wash and the machine did not work. She refused to go near the washing machine again.

Emotional memory is deeply personal. What is insignificant to one person may deeply resonate with the emotional memory of another. This is sometimes the reason that two people remember the same event differently, even though they were there together.

One family was shocked when their mother had forgotten the events of the morning of September 11, 2001 by the same afternoon. The person with dementia has no control over what they will or will not remember with their emotional memory. It is important to accept this and work around it. The common expression for this pattern of coping by family members is "going with the flow."

Some new emotionally mediated long-term memories are called 'latent' or 'implicit.' This means that we can see that the memory is obviously there, by the emotional reaction and actions of the person with dementia, but they are unable to recall it verbally. An example of this is given by Steven Sabat, in an article on implicit memory. A fellow with dementia, who was living at home with his wife, showed anger toward one of his sons. His wife had felt that it would be dangerous for her husband to continue to use the lawnmower; so he had asked her son to remove it, and told her husband what she had done. The anger he showed toward his son was in stark contrast to the loving, warm relationship they had previously enjoyed. This man, however, could not recall that his son had taken the lawnmower.

Another example of a latent emotional memory is that of two strangers who happened to live on the same nursing home unit. One day, for no apparent reason that anyone else could figure out, they started hitting each other every time they saw each other in the hall. The staff tried everything they could to encourage them to get along, but nothing worked. Perhaps they each reminded the other of someone they had known in the past, or they had an altercation that had not been witnessed by anyone else. No one ever figured out what started this behaviour. Eventually the staff decided to keep them from seeing each other, in the hopes that a lack of recurrence would help the emotional memory disappear for both of them. After five or six weeks, these two people did see each other accidentally. However, with all the time that had gone by, both had fortunately lost the memory of disliking the other, and the staff could let them wander freely within the unit again without having to help them avoid each other. Implicit or latent memories of recent events could account for a person with dementia crying, withdrawing or becoming hostile without being able to recall explain why they react that way.

In order to avoid reinforcing a negative emotional memory, I have often encouraged family members to avoid the topic of this memory altogether, if possible. Take for example, a person with dementia who tries a day program and is adamant about not returning. It is best to avoid the topic altogether for many weeks, rather than trying repeatedly to encourage and convince them to try it again. Once the memory fades, families are often able to reintroduce the day program later in a different way with successful results, and without the person remembering that they had disliked it in the past. The carers need to pursue getting the person with dementia into the day program in order to arrange respite for themselves.

If a person is spontaneously bringing up a negative emotional memory, such as the loss of a driver's licence, it is helpful to be mindful of their emotions. If their family member contradicts them, argues that the loss of the licence was justified, and attempts to convince them time and again, the emotions of the person with dementia will remain strong and negative. On the other hand, the family member could sympathize and validate their feelings in an understanding way (for example, "I don't blame you for being upset, it must be so difficult for you"). If after that they can gently guide the conversation away from the lost licence so they are distracted by a topic that creates positive emotions such as joy, delight and laughter, they may be able to ease the pain of this memory.

1.E. Procedural Memory

When people with dementia do the same thing over and over again, they will often form a new memory of that procedure. For example, a person who is admitted to a nursing home may need to be led from their room to the dining room and back, because they do not know the way. After a few months, they are able to get there on their own and find their own room again. They have slowly established a new long-term memory by repeating a procedure. Contrast this with establishing a procedural memory with the assistance of an intact short-term memory. When you are staying in a hotel, you may have difficulty finding your room the first time you go there, but the second time, you turn the correct way down the corridor and go to the approximate location of your room without thinking much about it.

The accidental establishment of a procedural memory was illustrated when a group of people with early dementia talked together, on one occasion, about not being able to recall the contents of the newspaper article they had just read. They each had the experience of reading a headline, thinking it was interesting, and then reading the article. Once they had finished reading the article, they realized that they couldn't remember a thing that it said. So they would read it again. After reading the same article five or six times, they would give up and move on to another article. They found it remarkable that all of them had experienced the same difficulty. They forgot the content of the articles, but had the procedural memory they had formed of trying over and over to remember what they read and their emotional experience of forgetting it. It was a relief for them to find that others had had the same experience and they had a good laugh.

The ability of people with dementia to establish new memories using their procedural memory has been actively researched. Cameron Camp and his associates at the Menorah Park Centre in Ohio have developed a method they call "Spaced Retrieval," which makes it possible for someone to help a person with dementia to develop new habits or procedures. This method allows the establishment of a procedural memory for a simple one-step task using carefully planned and researched training procedures repeated at specially spaced time intervals.

Paradoxically, people are able to develop new habits, such as using a walker correctly, but they do not remember being taught. This valuable new method is starting to make a difference to the daily lives of many people with early or middle stage dementia. It is quite evident to those who work in long-term care settings, that people with dementia are able to get accustomed to new procedures. Spaced Retrieval is a training process that allows others to formally access the retained ability of people with dementia to have new procedural learning (www.myersresearch.org).

It is human nature to teach someone how to do something when they cannot do it. If a person with dementia no longer recalls a person's name, they may have lost that memory permanently. Teaching them the name in an ordinary way, by expecting them to remember your instructions, will result in frustration for you and a sense of failure for them. If they can be taught using the method of spaced retrieval, they may be able to use the name with that person again, with your assistance. Research scientists are just beginning to explore the possibilities of teaching new or forgotten material to people with Alzheimer's disease, and there is hope of making an impact on their daily lives which may last for months or even a couple of years.

While spaced retrieval can help people learn, or relearn, simple, one-step tasks, it cannot reverse the loss of the ability to think rationally, to memorize, to think in the abstract, to have insight, to consider many facts at once in order to solve a problem, or to assess the feelings of one's own body and reach a conclusion about what one should do next in order to resolve difficulties.

Here are a few examples of families using procedural memory to help the person with dementia establish new habits. One family found that a fellow could drive well, but often became lost when he was out driving. He did not realize he had a problem, but they wanted him to stop driving for his own safety. His wife asked him once a week or so if it could be her turn to drive because her licence renewal was coming up and she needed to practise. She gradually increased the frequency of asking for her turn until she was doing the driving most of the time. Then, she started to automatically head for the driver's side of the car whenever they walked toward the car, without saying anything. After about six to eight weeks, her husband always went to the passenger side and never again expected to be the driver. She had helped him form a new procedural memory, which was that whenever he got into the car, he sat in the passenger seat. This was done without arguing and rationalizing that he should no longer drive. This non-confrontational approach to ceasing driving is positive, but not always possible.

Another fellow became lost in his new apartment building. He knew which floor he lived on, and that he and his wife lived in the first apartment on the right after getting out of the elevator. However, whenever he put the garbage down the chute at the end of the hall, he repeatedly went into the first apartment on the right on the way back, and ended up in someone else's place. He had formed an emotional memory and a procedural memory of going into the wrong apartment after putting out the garbage. This couple designed a procedural memory-training program together, and over the space of a few weeks, he was able to learn to get back to his own apartment after putting out the garbage. He was greatly relieved, as he had insight into his behaviour, and felt very badly whenever he suddenly and unexpectedly found himself in someone else's home.

One lady recounted a visit to her aunt. Her aunt didn't recognize her, but took her on a tour of the house. She passed by the stove and said, "You don't use this unless someone is with you." She passed by the back door and instructed, "You can't go out here unless you tell someone." You can see that this family successfully established these procedural memories by repeating them until they were new habits.

Often the procedural memories that are established are not complete. For example, a person with dementia may learn that a bus comes to take them to a place regularly, they go to a building where they have lots of fun and then they come home again. However, they cannot remember that they are going to an Alzheimer Day Away program, what address the building has, which days they attend, and the times that they go back and forth.

Sometimes the new procedural memories just get established by accident without anyone specifically trying to do so. If it is intentional, it is important to keep the mood and approach positive and upbeat, especially if they are having difficulty with something like getting used to going to a day program. If you scold and argue, a negative association will be established with going to the day program. On the other hand, if you smile, hug, and perhaps go out for a treat after each time they return, they may be more willing to participate.

People with dementia due to Alzheimer's disease rely on their procedural memories to maintain their functioning. Many families noted that their parent could manage quite well at home in their own kitchen, however, if they were moved or came to visit and were in a strange kitchen, they had suddenly lost their abilities to make meals. In fact, they were no longer able to use their procedural memories to find food in the refrigerator, find implements, pots, pans, plates and cutlery in the drawers. A similar issue can arise when the person with dementia is visiting a strange house and suddenly becomes incontinent. They may not be able to find the bathroom. At their own home, they have been able to use their procedural memory to always successfully locate the toilet without assistance. You may be able to relate to your own procedural memory if you think of what happens when you drive someone else's car. Your hands automatically go to the space where the controls are located in your car. You have to stop and think, and then you are able to orient yourself to the unfamiliar car.

One fellow was in the habit of driving to his daughter's place for supper each night. It was a matter of going a few blocks and he came every night on time without any reminders. He didn't show up one evening, and when his daughter called, he said he wasn't going to come. She drove to his place to check on him. On her way, she found that there was roadwork and she had to take a detour. She realized that he was able to drive to her place only if he took the same route all the time, but if he had to reason his way around a detour, he could not. He could not get to his daughter's house if he didn't follow the exact procedure he knew.

This story illustrates the difficulty that people with dementia have in adapting to change. They are relying on their procedural memory, and so not being able to use the same procedure stops them from continuing. Since their short-term memory is unavailable, they are unable to learn a new procedure quickly. In the previous story as well, the geographic disorientation, which will be discussed later, would also result in this fellow being unable to remember the map of the area in his mind sufficiently to figure out a new route. In order to solve the problem of finding a new route to his daughter's house, this fellow would have had to make three or four decisions about which way to turn on a few streets, hold all of those decisions in his mind as he thought about the new route he would take and then recall them in order as he made his way. This is a complex cognitive task, which requires an intact short-term memory, and so this type of problem solving is no longer available to a person whose short-term memory has been affected by their disease process.

Many times people have talked about their loved one in a nursing home, who for one reason or another, has been moved to a different room. Many months go by until they stop going into their old room. Adapting to the change of rooms means slowly undoing the old procedure and establishing a new one.

One lady told me that she was unhappy because her mother always reacted negatively when she came over. In contrast, when her brother would visit, her mother was always excited to see him and gave him a warm greeting. When I inquired about how their visits usually went, the daughter went on to explain that she usually made her mother's household arrangements and took her shopping and to appointments. She felt as though she was always having to 'lay down the law' to tell her mother what had to happen and how they needed to proceed. By contrast, her brother, although he also helped his mother a lot, made a habit of making his mother laugh by making faces at her, and he was generally jovial. My interpretation of this is that their mother made procedural memories of their visits. She would remember that her daughter would always be bossy and frowning and her son was always laughing. This daughter was looking forward to taking a lighter approach and inserting more laughter into her daily care for her mother. This is not an easy thing to do. The grief that family members feel naturally leads them to being sombre, sad and serious. The idea of joking around seems inappropriate. Regaining the ability to laugh is a great gift for everyone.

Thoughtful Dementia Care:
Understanding the Dementia Experience

Procedural memories that have been made before the onset of dementia are often available for many months or years after the diagnosis is made. There are many examples of this. One lady, although she could no longer knit by herself, was able to teach her daughter how to knit. She could concentrate on one particular knitting stitch at a time and pass this knowledge along. A fellow was no longer able to govern the family investments because he couldn't remember what transactions he had made. However, he was still able to tell his wife the procedure he had always used to evaluate what investments were sound and how to manage these from day to day. One lady could no longer sit independently, but if held up on a piano bench, could play the piano beautifully, to the enjoyment of all those around her. People, who can paint, may change their style, but still enjoy themselves. Drumming circles are very popular in many nursing home residences, and often the people with dementia who can no longer express themselves are delighted to use their old procedural memory of drumming. It is helpful for the person with dementia, if those who are caring for them remember what over-learned procedural skills they had when they were well, and give them the opportunity to be active using these skills, either independently or with some support.

2. Other Cognitive Changes

2.A. Insight

The ability to have insight is reliant on having intact brain cells in the area of the brain which functions to allow us to evaluate how we are doing. If that area of the brain is destroyed, the person will not be able to have insight into their own abilities. Most people with dementia that I have met or known about are in the middle of a spectrum, on a range between those who have no insight whatsoever and those who have a lot of insight. However, even those with a lot of insight did not seem to completely comprehend the full impact of the disease on their families and themselves.

If the person with dementia has an intact ability to have insight into their own behaviour, they will recognize that their memory and their abilities are poor. They will go off to get something, arrive in a room, and not remember why they went there and they will be upset by this. They may express anger when they come home without the items they were supposed to buy. They will experience frustration when they try to cut the grass and cannot remember how to start the lawnmower.

For the person whose insight has been destroyed by their disease process, things will not seem normal, but they may express it by blaming others for the things that are going wrong. They are feeling distress, are unaware of anything about themselves that may be causing the distress, and so they look elsewhere for the explanation. Their loss of the ability to realize that there is anything wrong with themselves is called anosognosia. These people are not 'in denial;' they honestly are not able to realize that they have a disease that is causing them problems, because the part of the brain that allows such reasoning has been damaged.

The people with insight are often able to discuss the fact that they have Alzheimer's disease or whichever disease is causing their dementia, and the difficulties they have associated with it. They may become depressed and they may grieve as they grapple with the enormity of their diagnosis. These people may need help with their depressive symptoms, possibly including medication. People with dementia who have their insight intact are also able to benefit from education and support in the form of professionally led group discussions of the emotions that they are experiencing; and, discussing as a group any issues that they raise.

People without insight, on the other hand, will deny adamantly that anything is wrong, because they are no longer capable of recognizing what is happening to themselves. They will not come to groups for people with dementia because they are certain there is nothing the matter with them and they don't belong in such a group. They trust their memory and therefore feel that if their lives are 'topsy-turvy,' someone else is responsible, because they have no memory of causing the difficult situations themselves. They have a short-term memory loss, so they do not remember that people have told them they are coming to visit, or to take them shopping, or that they have a doctor's appointment. The continual repetition of being surprised by events that they are expected to participate in, promotes the development of a procedural memory. The procedural memory for how everyone treats them is that they are never told anything, and that they are always expected to come on outings without warning. On the other hand, people who still have their insight will form a procedural memory that they are always forgetting that people have called or have said they are coming to visit.

One example of a person without insight is a woman whose family was taking her across the ocean for a visit to her former home and her extended family. Her children told her a dozen times a day about this trip as it approached. When they got to the airport, she angrily said to them, "What do you think I am, a child? Why didn't you tell me about this trip?" This illustrates the blaming on others for the situation when the person cannot comprehend that they are doing the forgetting themselves.

A fellow who retained his language skills into the late stage gave his family a glimpse of his thoughts when he no longer had insight into the basic elements of his context. He was sitting in the nursing home lounge beside his wife, who had come to visit. Across the room from them was a lady who resembled her in body shape and hairstyle, and both wore glasses. Her husband leaned toward his wife, pointed at the woman across the room and asked: "Is that you over there?" Having had years of experience of similarly startling revelations, she calmly replied, "No, but she looks like me, doesn't she?"

The complex cognitive activity of insight is not something that can be relearned. On occasion, I was asked by family members to convince the person with dementia that they actually had Alzheimer's or a similar disease. I always replied that it is impossible to do so when the person no longer has their insight. The changes in their brain make it impossible for them to comprehend and remember this information. If a person has a disease such as cancer or diabetes, they are able to change their behaviour to adapt to life with the new illness. However, it is their brain that gives them the ability to adapt. When the brain is diseased, there is no other body organ that can take over and give back the insight or decide to make allowances for the brain's forgetfulness. This sounds obvious, however, I have met many people who have never thought about everything their brain does for them and what the consequences are when the brain is not functioning.

When a person has insight into their inability to remember things, they sometimes seem to continuously try to 'kick start' their memory by almost obsessing on a future event. For example, if they are told there is a doctor's appointment coming up, they may frequently verbalize the worry that they should be leaving for it, or the worry that they may have missed it. They may do this many times a day, for many days, until the appointment. Often, family carers wait until such appointments are quite near to tell the person with dementia about them, and thus help them both avoid stress.

Lack of insight on the part of the person with dementia can cause them to create arguments. Trying to avoid arguing back will prevent the situation from escalating, and will help both of you enjoy less stress. If you are arguing constantly with the person with dementia, they may develop a procedural memory that being with you is unpleasant. It is helpful in your relations with the person with dementia to be conscious of establishing a positive and happy procedural memory of your interaction.

For example, perhaps every time you go home after shopping, your wife with dementia scolds you for having been away for hours and not telling her where you were going. In reality, you were actually gone for about an hour and you told her six times you were going to the grocery store and you have groceries in your arms. She no longer has the insight to realize that you have probably told her and she forgot. You start to cringe at the thought of walking in the door because you know that you will get a very angry greeting.

It is important for you to try to take control of this repeated event. Instead of going in the door with your head down waiting for the harsh words from her, plant a big smile on your face; tell her you are so glad to be home, that you missed her and that you love her very much. Bring her a treat. Slowly, her habit of greeting you with anger will disappear and she will respond to your positive approach.

I have frequently called this method 'aggressive friendliness.' People with dementia have lost sight of the context of your relationship. It helps them to understand if you show your warmth and love very openly with smiles and cheerful conversation. If you feel as if you are exaggerating your expression of positive emotions, you are actually expressing yourself in an appropriate way for a person with dementia to understand your message.

People who still have their insight are often able to help keep themselves safe. One lady would go on walks, but never lose sight of her daughter's house. She had formed an emotional memory from one incident in which she was lost for an hour and needed help to get back home. On one occasion, this same woman would agree to go to a musical play in another city, only if her name and address and that of her daughter were pinned on her coat; she had enough insight into her illness to know she wouldn't be able to get herself home if they became separated in the crowd.

In contrast, a gentleman who lacked insight would often leave home to go running. He had no concept that he could become lost. Since he was a former marathon runner, he could cover quite a distance in a short time. The family had to follow him in the car, trying to convince him to get in and come home. After trying many approaches, they had to put up a solid fence. When he could no longer see the road, it didn't occur to him to go for a run. At the same time, he could still enjoy the fresh air in the yard.

Each individual has unique needs. People with insight need more support for their depression, fears and high anxiety. People without insight need more support for their safety, and understanding when they blame others for their mistakes and misunderstandings.

2.B. Judgement

In order to make good judgements we require accuracy in our memory, perceptions, language, and in our interpretation and understanding of the context of the situation. The enormous changes in these cognitive skills with dementia lead to changes in the ability to use judgement as the person has used it in the past. A person with dementia may not be able to take everything into account when they make a judgement, and may forget many important factors when making a decision.

Think about yourself making a decision to buy a car. You have to evaluate how much you can afford to pay, when you need to get the car, whether you want two or four doors, whether it will be new or used, how the guidebooks rank the different models and years, whether it will be a van or a sedan, what colour you prefer, and many other factors. In order to reach a decision, you need to hold all of this information in your mind at the same time. If you only have one component of the problem in your mind, as people with short-term memory loss do, since they can only think about one thing at a time, your decision is likely to be faulty.

Take for instance the fellow who went out and ordered a new car at a dealer. He bought the same one his neighbour had bought because he admired it, and that was the only factor he took into consideration. He was no longer supposed to drive. He took the car keys when his wife was in the bathtub and drove to the car dealership, and that, in itself, was a faulty decision. He was told not to drive when he was diagnosed with Vascular Dementia, and his driving was unsafe. He remembered that he wasn't supposed to drive, but it made him angry, so at times he drove anyway. This couple had a good car that was less than a year old and they didn't need and couldn't afford a second car. His wife found out about it only when the dealer called to say they couldn't get the colour he wanted. Fortunately, they were understanding and cancelled the contract.

An inability to exercise judgement can result in financial difficulties, if the person with dementia is not able to accurately decide whether they need something or whether they can afford it. Many people found that the person with dementia would amass huge credit card bills and make other financial decisions that were detrimental to them. One lady spontaneously gave away a lot of money to a wealthy relative. She was thinking of a time when this person was much younger and she had helped her. Another person used an inheritance to purchase a house, and then forgot that he had spent the money and needed his family's help to reorganize his debts. A fellow had his storage unit for his apartment stuffed with dozens of shirts, still in their store wrappers. He insisted on buying a new one whenever they went to the mall.

Forgetting all the steps of a procedure can lead to faulty judgement when it comes to paying for things in a store. People forget why they have to go to the cash register and how to line up once they get there. They may go into the store, find the item they want and leave. Our local police had a policy of asking to see the person's wandering registry card as proof that dementia was the reason they had left the store without paying for something.

Many people with dementia, who are unable to make wise decisions about their property, have money fraudulently taken from them by dishonest friends and relatives. Preventing this possibility takes careful planning before the onset of dementia. In Canada, it is a criminal offence to use a Power of Attorney for your own interest to the detriment of the person with dementia. When anyone chooses the person they want to be their power of attorney, or decision-maker, they should choose the one or two amongst their family members that they trust the most, and who have a good track record in managing their own money and property. Setting limits on what the person who is the power of attorney can do with their assets is useful as well. Such limits might be, for example, stipulating that their assets must stay only in their own name; that their investments can be reinvested, but not sold; that their income, assets, and any proceeds of their assets are to be used only for their living expenses and are not to be loaned to any family member; that there must be open accounting for all in the family to inspect; and, the conditions under which the power of attorney may be activated, are useful limitations. Powers of attorney are very useful to make arrangements in the care of the person with dementia go smoothly, however good legal counsel is advisable when arranging them.

The lack of judgement shown by the person with dementia may also result in severe embarrassment for the family. One fellow, who had been a very proper gentleman all his life, unzipped and urinated into the river in a public park with many people nearby. He was oblivious to the scandal he had created, and, although there had been signs of memory loss, this incident helped the family realize that there was something seriously wrong. Another lady lacked judgement when her husband took her into the family bathroom at their church. She needed his help with her clothing, and also he couldn't leave her on her own, as she would get lost easily. Once she was finished, he decided he'd better use the facilities while he had the chance. He could not stop her when she left, leaving the door wide open with the whole congregation milling around and he was acutely embarrassed. Fortunately, others jumped to their rescue. Both of these incidents of poor judgement resulted from the person with dementia being able to think about only one thing at a time.

This type of behaviour may also be termed 'disinhibition.' It is the result of multiple losses in cognition affecting the person's ability to exercise their usual standard of judgement. When we are out in public, we stop ourselves from acting in ways that would be embarrassing to ourselves and to others, or that would be unacceptable or even illegal in our society. When we do this we are 'inhibiting' our behaviour. We are making judgements about what is proper behaviour and acting on those judgements. When people with dementia are acting in an improper manner, they are no longer inhibited; they are disinhibited.

Disinhibition can have a positive or a negative effect, or somewhere in between. For example, one woman was a grandmother many times over and had taught school in the early grades during her career. She had always behaved very properly towards children. After she developed dementia, she would go to the street in front of the local school when the children were to be dismissed. She would talk to them and hug them, which was certainly not acceptable. She was disinhibited in terms of her expression of affection for the children. She was unable to understand that this was wrong, and unable to learn to stop. Another instance was a woman in the early stage of dementia, who had always kept secret the abortion she had before she met the man she married, but became disinhibited and began to talk about it and to cry about the child she had lost. Because of the circumstances she described, her husband realized it was not likely that she was making up the story. He realized that if he had known about it at the time, he never would have married her. However, he loved her dearly and cherished all the fifty plus years they had been together. He said, "I know no one can do anything about this, but I just need someone to witness what I am experiencing." Another example was the fellow who had always inhibited himself from talking to his children about his very difficult childhood and his wartime experiences. When he developed dementia, he was no longer able to inhibit himself and started to talk to his son about his life. His son had always wanted to know, and very much appreciated having a better understanding of his father. He felt that the dementia had brought them closer together.

The inability to exercise judgement in daily life is often seen in the confusion that people show when they are trying to decide what to wear. There are so many factors to consider when you look into a closet of clothes to decide what to put on: the weather, where you are going, what matches, what you recently wore. People with dementia, who are having difficulty with these choices, often either put on clothing that is inappropriate or they fail to get dressed at all, and spend the day in their pyjamas. This is when families need to start helping to narrow the choices, so the person with dementia is assisted with the decision-making that they can no longer do.

One lady laid out her husband's clothes on the bed and left him to get himself dressed as she did every morning. After half an hour she went back upstairs to see what was keeping him so long. By accident, she had left two belts on the bed and she found him going back and forth between the brown

Thoughtful Dementia Care:
Understanding the Dementia Experience

belt and the black belt, unable to decide which to put on. Even such seemingly inconsequential decision-making tasks may become impossible for some people with dementia.

Lack of judgement by the person with dementia can also create great merriment in the family. This happened in one family when the fellow with dementia, a husband, father, grandfather and formerly a very proper church elder, patted the bottom of the lady in front of him, a stranger, in his impatience to move faster up the church aisle to get communion. His wife later apologized and explained the circumstances. The laughter this created in the family bound them together, gave them strength, and made them cherish 'Dad' even more. However, his wife carried a card in her purse, which said, "The person I am with has dementia. Please smile and include them in our conversation." She was able to show this discreetly if a lapse in judgement by her husband created awkwardness and she was unable to explain the situation in front of him.

Even though the person with dementia may act in a way that causes some embarrassment when they attend their place of worship, it is often comforting for them to continue attending. They are likely able to feel quite comfortable during a service, which follows the same procedure as the hundreds of other services they have attended, and will feel the belonging and the meaning that their religion has always given them. Others in the community need to encourage the person and their carer to come, in order to be supportive and help to decrease the isolation of the couple, which so often accompanies dementia.

Having others understand that the person with dementia has difficulty with judgement and decision-making can be very supportive to their carer. One woman described going into a hardware store with her husband, who was very early in his dementia and still trying to do some projects around the house. The clerk became annoyed with the length of time her husband was taking to make his choice. She was able to quietly tell him about the dementia without her husband overhearing. Immediately, the clerk changed his whole attitude. He slowed down, and went step by step to help her husband pick exactly what he needed. She was so grateful for this understanding that, days later, when she told about it, her smile was still radiant. Often carers feel alone in their efforts to support the person with dementia, and a little help from others makes an enormous difference to them.

2.C. Emotions

The ability to feel emotions stays fairly intact in the person with dementia. They continue to feel the whole array of emotions: happiness, sadness, joy, grief, anger, puzzlement, anxiety, contentment, hurt, embarrassment, discomfort, fear, disgust, insecurity, resentment, pleasure, and so on.

One thing that changes is the amount of control people with dementia have of the way they express what they are feeling. People who have no dementia can sit in a room and feel a strong emotion, such as anger or joy, but hide it from anyone else. No one knows how they feel, and they can control what they say to soften the expression of that emotion. However, this type of control is no longer available as dementia progresses. If a person with dementia becomes angry, they may respond immediately, even though in the past they would have been able to contain an angry response. Some people view this as a personality change, but it is more easily understood and accepted as a lack of judgement resulting from the dementia.

Control requires thinking about at least two things at once: how we are feeling; and, how our response will affect those who are listening to us. Because many people with dementia are not able to simultaneously think about what they want to say and what its effect will be on the person they say it to, they may make hurtful statements such as, "I hate that orange coat you're wearing," or "My goodness, you have put on so much weight," which can hurt the feelings of the person to whom they are talking.

People caring for those with dementia need to become resilient to such comments and learn to refrain from taking them personally. When comments are made by the person with dementia that are very insulting about another person's character, some family members think that the person with dementia has always felt that way about them, and just not said it until now. I don't believe this to be true. I feel that if the person who now has dementia has always been admiring and positive in the past towards a person, that is the true measure of how they felt. A person with dementia may have negative emotions churning inside them much of the time, especially if they are living in stressful circumstances. Living in that state unfortunately can give them a tendency to talk about others in a very negative way. It's almost as though they have the feeling overwhelm them first, and afterward, they look for a reason for feeling the way they do, and then mistakenly blame someone else for treating them badly. It is very difficult, for a child especially, to accept that a grandparent cannot control their tendency to making accusations that are not the truth. This takes many months of patient explaining by other adults in the household.

Emotional tensions can run high in a household where an older person with dementia tries to enforce rules for the children which were appropriate one or two generations ago and is unable to stop doing so. Helping the children learn how to establish strong patterns of warmth and friendliness in their interactions with their grandparent will permit them to use distraction methods similar to those their parents use. The children in the family often enjoy simple games with their grandparent with dementia such as tossing a ball into a laundry basket. It is a good idea to shift the focus of the children from the difficulties they are having with their grandparent with dementia, to attempts to be upbeat by, for example, having a contest to see "who can get Grandpa to laugh?"

The person with short-term memory loss is thinking about one thing for a short period, and then when they are distracted, they think about something else. If there are strong emotions associated with these thoughts, they may appear to be having mood swings, especially, for example, if they change from thinking about something that makes them very sad to thinking about something that makes them feel happy. Many families described the mood swings that happened after an argument or an unpleasant event. Fifteen minutes later, the carer would still be upset, but the person with dementia no longer remembered the incident and might be quite cheerful. For people with a close bond, such as a married couple, this would represent yet another instance of no longer sharing the journey of their lives. The well spouse is left to deal with the emotional aftermath alone, while the spouse with dementia does not remember the event. One woman described the sadness and guilt she felt as she sensed herself becoming emotionally separated from her husband. She was going through an emotional shift of being part of 'us,' she and her husband, to being 'me,' herself alone.

Without dementia, we can usually change our own emotions by doing something different. A person who is feeling sad and depressed can take a walk, do some cleaning, do chores such as cutting the grass or shovelling the snow, in order to distract themselves from their negative feelings and get physical exercise to help themselves feel happier. If someone feels angry, they can calm themselves down and think of all the reasons it would be better not to express their anger in order to keep their friends or have good relations in their family. They think of some other way to rectify an unjust situation in their close relationships. All of this active thought requires an intact short-term memory to hold all the factors open for mental evaluation at once and to evaluate the repercussions of each possible response. People with dementia lose the capacity to problem solve their way out of such dilemmas.

You can assist the person with their emotions. The person with dementia, particularly late in the disease, lives in the moment, without a context. They are without a perceived past or future. If you help them enjoy the moment, it is a gift of positive emotions. Your gift of laughter or pleasure can result in a positive mood that lasts for hours. Laughter at some of the comical situations you will experience is healthy and to be shared with the person with dementia by hugging them, or somehow showing that the two of you have shared a special moment. Carers can also help by intentionally distracting people with dementia in order to help them improve their mood. In the early stages the distraction should be slow, subtle and perhaps open. You may say "We're feeling upset. Let's listen to some music to help us feel better." I do mean to use the word 'we.' If the person with dementia is upset, the carer will be also. The approach is unique to each individual and each carer has to discover the best approach and then continuously evaluate its effectiveness and change it as the person's dementia progressively worsens.

Sometimes a sudden distraction is necessary. One fellow, upset about taking so many pills, grabbed his wife's arm to prevent her from helping him take his pills. He had always been a gentle person, but because of his lack of judgement, he was hurting her arm. She knew about using distraction, so she turned and pointed and said, "Look at that bird out the window!" Of course, being able to think about only one thing at a time, he dropped her arm and went to the window. "I don't see any bird," he replied. "Oh, dear! It must have flown away," she answered. Then she waited for a couple of hours before she cautiously approached him to take his pills again. People with dementia often forget why they are taking the pills, and many, like this gentleman, become impatient about taking them. If the pills upset their stomach, or have an unpleasant aftertaste, they may build a procedural memory that taking the pills causes problems. If they cannot remember why they are taking the pills, they may even conclude that they are being poisoned. Many carers ask the doctor to eliminate all but the most essential medications, to avoid the emotional stress that taking them can cause.

People with short-term memory loss are no longer able to carefully evaluate their behaviour, nor are they able to take decisive steps to move themselves from a negative mood to a positive mood. They may stay in a bad mood long after they have forgotten the incident that inspired that mood. They need people around them who are resilient to hurtful comments, and who are able to choose a solution to a negative emotion and help them work their way to a more positive emotional state. Carers gain in strength and ability as they try approaches, one after the other, and settle on the approach that works best for that time.

It is important to realize the effect you have on the emotions of the person with dementia. They are extremely sensitive to your body language, and the tone of voice you use when you speak. They may easily react with anxiety to a frown on your face or tension in your voice. As you develop an awareness of their reaction to your moods, you will become adept at being sure you are not communicating anxiety. If you do upset them, take a few minutes to gather your thoughts, calm down, and then try again with a distraction or a different approach.

Usually we are not aware of our body language, unless we have had special training in using it. Notice what it is you do when you are feeling agitated, upset, in pain, angry or frustrated. These are the emotions in you to which the person with dementia is most likely to react. I believe that when a person with dementia senses these emotions in their carer, it makes them feel insecure. They are not able to remember what it is you are reacting to, if it is something other than their behaviour. Usually they take any negative emotion you demonstrate in a personal way. If you are upset because someone cut you off in traffic, they may feel that you are angry with them, even though they had nothing to do with the incident. People with dementia do best if they are in a quiet, predictable environment as they can use their procedural memory to understand what is happening. If your emotions are volatile, they are uncertain what to do, and they feel unsafe and may become afraid.

If a person with dementia is continually exposed to someone else losing their temper, they have a great deal of difficulty remaining calm. This type of situation provokes uncertainty and anxiety and they may react by behaving as though they need to defend themselves. The person with dementia cannot adapt to the changing moods of their carer, especially negative moods. Part of thoughtful dementia care is to recognize this and to try to minimize your expression of negative emotions in their presence.

Perhaps because they are losing their spoken language, people with dementia seem to be more sensitive to the body language of those around them than they were when they were well. Many people have commented that their family member with dementia understood when the carer was upset, sometimes even before the carer realized it themselves. This is particularly true in the early stage.

If there is an incident in which the person with dementia seems to suddenly react badly with their behaviour and language, try to review in your mind what has happened in the past half-hour or so. If this happens frequently, you may want to write down what you notice. Sometimes, there is a pattern that emerges which was not visible before the circumstances were written down, and then examined to see if there is any theme. For example, the person with dementia may get upset at different times on a few different days of the week. By keeping track of what is happening, you may discover that their mood changes about ten minutes after you have been down in the basement doing laundry. You might be able to help them by taking them to the basement with you and giving them a one-step task that they can do to help with the work. If they are not able to go to the basement, putting on some music or a recording of your voice telling a story may help. If you can't find any solution, you may need to consider finding someone to help occupy the person with dementia or someone to help you with the laundry. This doesn't have to be paid help. I met two ladies, who took their friend with dementia out for lunch at the same time every week. Her husband could use that time to bank, shop, do housework, or make an appointment with the doctor for himself and be certain of being able to get there. This is when you take people up on the offer of "let me know if there's anything I can do to help." Being able to get things done yourself to stay organized will help you emotionally, and therefore help the person with dementia remain calm and secure. Accepting help from outside the family unit is very difficult to do, however, decreasing the stress on the carer helps prolong the time that the person with dementia can be cared for at home. The book, "Share the Care," by Capossela and Warnock, describes a formal method of setting up a community of support around a person with a terminal illness.

If the person with dementia is reacting badly for no apparent reason, it is best not to cause further stress to them by asking what's wrong or demanding an explanation. I have often encouraged carers to remove themselves briefly (for ten to thirty minutes), as long as the person with dementia is safe. Say something like "Oops! I have to go to the bathroom, I'll be right back." Rest quietly for a few minutes, calm yourself down and try to figure out what in the environment or in your behaviour made the person upset. It may be neither – many people with dementia have upsetting misunderstandings and also perhaps hallucinations. Coping with hallucinations will be discussed in the section entitled "Delusions, Illusions and Hallucinations." Careful listening and observing will help you.

The bathroom is a refuge for many carers. I frequently got whispered phone calls from carers in the bathroom trying to figure out what to do next. They were in the bathroom with the door locked, the phone in the bathtub and the shower curtains pulled, trying to keep the person with dementia from hearing what they were saying. Often they made calls to family members in this way. People with dementia very frequently become agitated when their carer is on the telephone. It could be that they feel they are being talked about. Since they have dementia and are a great concern to all family members, this is often true. The person with dementia feels anxiety, fear, embarrassment and shame when they know that they are being talked about. Even if they are not the topic of conversation, they may think they are. The patience of a person with dementia waiting for their carer to get off the phone is very limited, especially when they need help just to occupy their own time. Putting the phone call on the speaker so they can also hear and talk may help. The main carer does need to talk. If others visit in pairs, one can visit with the person with dementia and the other can visit with the carer. It is important to seek out what you need.

Fear and anxiety are the dominant emotions that people with dementia feel, when they are not deliberately helped to feel calm and secure. Since they usually cannot remember the context of their environment, the people with them, nor what will be happening next, they can feel very nervous and unsafe. Diseases that cause dementia remove all the psychological anchors in a person's life. Think of how you would feel if you could not recognize the room or the place you are standing in, who the person is who is talking to you, what year it is, what is happening now and what will be happening next. With their procedural memory, they are able to know that they are in this situation quite frequently. This would make anyone feel extremely insecure, anxious, and, at times, terrified. Whenever a person is reacting in a negative way, assume that they are anxious about something, even if you cannot figure out what it is. Respond in a soothing, calming manner, showing with your body language and your facial expression that you are a friend who means them no harm.

A person with dementia, who lacks emotional control and also lacks judgement about appropriate responses, may strike out if they feel threatened. Almost always, this occurs as a result of the person with dementia thinking that they have to defend themselves. Knowing what circumstances increase a person's fear and anger, and helping them to avoid those circumstances, can greatly lower the chance of physical violence. For example, one fellow who had dementia and diabetes would frequently go to the refrigerator for extra food. His wife, who was his carer, would argue with him and scold him, and she began to physically wrestle the food out of his hands. This made him angry. He was quite a bit bigger and stronger than she was, and if the physical struggles had escalated, she could have been hurt. I encouraged her to stop this approach immediately. Not every aspect of health can be perfectly regulated when a person has dementia, especially if they are uncooperative. In this case, it was better to alter his insulin to lower his resulting high blood sugar, than it would have been to escalate the combat between them.

Another example is that of a fellow who was in bed complaining that he was cold. The carer felt the sheets and discovered that they were wet. She got dry sheets and then returned to the bed and removed the covers to get him up and change the sheets. He hit her arm. This was a fellow who had never hit anyone before. If you think about this situation carefully, you will realize that she had made a leap of logic that he was unable to make. She knew the sheets were wet and that in order for him to feel warm, they had to be changed. He knew that he was feeling cold and when she took off the covers, he felt colder. He felt the need to defend himself. Because of the dementia, he could no longer automatically follow her thinking and cooperate. She needed to give a slow, careful explanation of what she was going to do, step by step. This might include wrapping him in a blanket to meet his immediate need to be warmer. Watching his reaction with each step would let the carer know if he has sufficient understanding of the situation at that moment to cooperate and help her fix the situation.

The changes that a person with dementia experiences can lead to them feeling anxiety, fear and sometimes terror, as they lose their memory anchors to the reality of the world around them. Generally speaking, thoughtful dementia care means trying to keep people feeling calm and secure in their environment. Each person will have unique needs in what will help them stay calm and content.

Sometimes the change in context due to their long-term memory loss combines with a current situation to create stress for the person with dementia. For example, one fellow in a nursing home became very agitated every day about 4 P.M. In order to try to understand the cause, someone stayed with him from 3:30 to 4:30 P.M. to see what he was experiencing. The volunteers, activity staff and the day shift of nurses left at 4 P.M., and the evening shift went into report. The unit suddenly changed from a bustling hive of activity to the quiet of a deserted library. As it became quieter, the fellow with dementia began to pace and shout, "Who's on that line? Why aren't they working?" The things he was saying reflected the themes of a workplace. At one point in his working life he had been a factory supervisor. In his mind, he was back in that time, in that workplace. His interpretation of the sudden silence and lack of activity in his current environment was linked in his mind to his former workplace and he took the absence of activity to mean that the work on the factory line had ceased and he felt agitated and responsible to get it going again. His time context was verified by taking him to a mirror, pointing to his reflection, and asking him "Who is that?" He replied, "I don't know." Then he was shown a picture of himself taken fifty-five years earlier. "Who is this?" He was asked. He replied scornfully, looking at the person asking the questions as though they were quite dim-witted and couldn't see what was obvious, "That's me in my uniform, of course!"

It is important to validate the emotions of the person with dementia and to recognize that their emotions are real and appropriate in their reality. Listening carefully to the person with dementia and knowing their history are valuable tools to helping them. Trying to tell him that he is not in the factory is quite likely to increase his agitation, because in his reality as he understands it, that's exactly where he is. Giving him a reasonable explanation as to why the activity on the line has decreased (for example, "it's quitting time") is respectful of the context he thinks he is in, and of the reality he feels he is in at the moment. Ideally, this individual would benefit from a guided activity at that time, to prevent his agitation from being triggered by the staffing shift change.

Over years of working with people with dementia and their families, I developed an understanding that there is an angst that often accompanies dementia. People with this emotional disquietude are constantly searching for their lives to be normal again. The angst is about needing to know where they are, what they should be doing next and to be able to do it. It is about needing to feel that they are in the place where they belong and with the people they feel close to, that they are at home and at peace with themselves. Many people seemed uncomfortable in their own house, and these were the people who seemed to be very concerned that they could no longer care for their home as they once did. Just being at home made them restless and they were much happier being out for a drive. When they were out, there was no reminder of how much knowledge and ability they had lost, whereas when they were at home, there were reminders everywhere they looked. Not feeling safe also adds to this angst. One family had moved their mother four times over a single year, until they realized that her repeated unhappiness with the place in which she was living, was coming from her inability to feel at home anywhere. Another lady lived next door to her childhood home on a farm. When she asked to "go home," her family took her there. This did not satisfy her. Home is not a place; it is a feeling. As an approach to caring for people with dementia, helping them to feel at home, that they are welcome and they belong and are cherished, is a powerful and thoughtful method of care. When a person with dementia feels calm and secure, they can exist in a state of carefree contentment.

People who have dementia are also losing their ability to enjoy their lives as they had made them up to that point. They lose control over what they can do independently. They lose their understanding of their situation, their usefulness and their ability to be an equal in a relationship. Emotional distress and anxiety are to be expected. It is very legitimate for the person with dementia to be emotionally distraught over losing something like their driver's licence. Since they cannot keep in their minds why they have lost it, they can remain incensed and feeling cheated for a long time. Arguing with them that it is right that they no longer drive may not be helpful. Expressing sympathy and understanding, and reassuring them that they will be supported may be a more soothing response. The loss of independence is a legitimate cause of grief, and consolation is needed. Resolving grief takes longer for a person with dementia, and they need help.

As the disease becomes more advanced, people with dementia become unable to express their emotions with their facial muscles, or it may not occur to them to hug. They may respond negatively to the noise and confusion of many people present, as they are overwhelmed. This often happens at large family gatherings. A series of one-on-one visits in an adjacent room may be more tolerable. Young children, particularly, need to be given an explanation that "Grandpa still cares, he just can't show it." Even though a person shows very little expression, it is important to try to include them if they are able to tolerate the activity. Don't assume that it has no meaning to them. I remember one incident in a long-term care setting that taught me this lesson. It was Christmas time and one of the family members was dressed as Santa Claus, handing out little gifts to each resident. 'Santa' went to a few rooms to visit people who were not well enough to come to the resident lounge for the festivities. One lady had not spoken, smiled or even looked at anyone in over a year. However, when Santa came in, she smiled and burst into tears. Everyone felt touched by her response.

Helping a person remain calm and secure may mean making it easy for them to stay with you at all times. Many people with dementia feel insecure when they are alone and will follow their carer everywhere, a habit that has been called 'shadowing.' Sometimes they follow so closely that their carer bumps into them if they take a step backwards. Trying to convince them to go into another room will cause great stress to the person with dementia who experiences fear when they cannot see their carer.

Many people with dementia enjoy increased feelings of security when they are hugged, or someone holds their hand or sits so close that their arms are touching. Even people, who have never demonstrated affection by hugging or wanting to be hugged, may respond well. However, this is different from one individual to the next, and carers need to refrain if a person with dementia responds negatively to being touched.

Some people with dementia develop obsessions that continue for weeks, months or even years. It is as though all the fear and anxiety, which is building due to their losses of knowledge, ability and understanding, becomes focussed on one thought, which the person with dementia expresses many times a day with great agitation. For example, one woman was convinced that her neighbours had stolen the million dollars she had won. What she had seen was an advertising letter that gave her the chance to win a million dollars, and she mistakenly assumed she already had. Another woman became obsessed with packing for a family holiday. For three weeks after she found out they were going, she had clothes and open suitcases all over the furniture and the floors of every room in the house. She would pack, fold, unfold and repack all day long. Fortunately, this obsession ended when the holiday finally arrived. Lasting obsessions fade as the dementia progresses. Sometimes a person's obsession can be channelled into harmless activity. Someone who is worried about mail, for example, may be content to sort and organize the same box of flyers repeatedly.

The family of one lady with dementia did not interfere while she rearranged all of her dishes every day. They were on tables, or chairs, or the floor, or anywhere she could find a spot for them; and, she constantly moved them from one place to another. She was living on her own. Her family made sure her basic care was attended to, and since she wasn't harming anyone and appeared content, was facilitated to continue her obsessive activity.

Another fellow hoarded food in his room in a retirement home. With careful observation two things became apparent. Firstly, he was unable to get the saran wrap off the snacks that were brought to him; his fingers were no longer able to perform the fine movements needed, and his vision was not adequate to see where the edges of the saran wrap were, to start to peel it away from the food. Secondly, his hoarding was meeting his need to feel secure in the knowledge that he would always find something to eat. Some of it was taken away, but also some was left, so that he would not be deprived of the source of his security. Obsessions are usually present because they meet an emotional need for the person with dementia. It is important to try to uncover what the need is and help them meet it in a more socially acceptable manner.

Meeting the emotional needs of the person with dementia is more difficult for family members who have been abused, physically, financially or psychologically, by the person with dementia, in the past, before the dementia developed. Needing to give dementia care tends to bring up all the old unresolved issues in the family. Many times, carers needed to go into counselling themselves, because they needed to resolve their feelings about the issues of the past in order to stop experiencing the emotional upheaval that delivering care to their former abuser was causing. Some were able to suppress or resolve those issues in order to give direct care to the person with dementia. Others were not able to do so. Personally giving care for a family member with dementia should be voluntary. It is law in Canada that adult children have a duty of care to their incapable parents. Many family members were relieved when I pointed out they need not deliver the care themselves, but could arrange for the care to be delivered by others, without visiting or giving the hands-on care themselves.

Family members who had been abusive up until the time they developed dementia didn't necessarily stay that way. Often there was a personality change. A couple of people said that they felt the person with dementia somehow sensed that they needed to change their behaviour in order to continue to receive care in the family. It is embarrassing for the family member who has been abused to admit it. This makes it very difficult for them to share the problems they are having. Family members in this situation need to realize that their needs are important and legitimate and it is alright to give as much priority to caring for themselves as caring for the person with dementia, or seeing that they receive the care they need.

2.D. Abstract Thought

The thinking processes also change because abstract thought becomes difficult, and then impossible. People with dementia tend to think and talk about very concrete things, such as what is going on around them at the moment, as a result. Abstract concepts, such as numbers and arithmetic, become difficult early in the disease. Many people with dementia can no longer remember what a number represents and how to use numbers generally. One example of this was a fellow who tried to put up a new shelf in the laundry room. He had been very handy, able to fix and make almost anything around the house. However, when he tried to mount this new shelf, he found things had changed. He put up the brackets to support the shelf easily, and then measured the distance between them. He cut the board, only to discover that he had cut it too long. He measured again and trimmed off the excess, but discovered that the shelf was now far too short. He had lost his ability to work with numbers.

Difficulty dealing with abstract thought and numbers leads to difficulty with money management. Very often, one of the first indicators of a dementing process is mismanagement of finances and an inability to add and subtract in order to manage a chequebook or bank accounts. When combined with the deficit in short-term memory, this may result in debts not being paid, or being paid many times over. Often, people with Alzheimer's disease will pay for purchases with a bill or two, ask if it is enough, and trust that they are receiving the correct change. It is difficult, but important, for family to be sure that the person is not being taken advantage of by another who does not have their best interests at heart, or is working for their own personal advantage, rather than protecting the interests and assets of the person with dementia.

Another indicator that a person is having difficulty with abstract thought is they may no longer understand metaphors. You may say something like "a bird in the hand is worth two in the bush," meaning "it's better to have it than not have it." Rather than understand what you mean, the person with dementia who is having difficulty with abstract thought, may look around to see where the birds and the bushes are that you are talking about. Their thinking is very concrete. Since jokes are often based on metaphor and leaps of logic, people who are having difficulty using abstract thought are often not able to understand them.

That's not to say a person with dementia loses their sense of humour. Many people keep their good sense of humour for years, even poking fun at themselves. One fellow I saw fairly regularly for a time always told the same joke. "Every morning I read the obituaries, and if my name isn't there, I know it's going to be a good day!" I began to eagerly anticipate him telling this joke. His infectious laughter lit up the room.

2.E. Geographic Disorientation

Dementia also results in an inability to recognize one's surroundings and to find the way to a destination. In this case, long-term memory loss combines with changes in spatial abilities and short-term memory loss to contribute to geographic disorientation. The person may no longer be able to use their long-term memory to identify where they currently live. They may have lost their ability to use their sense of direction in a familiar environment. Their short-term memory loss may prevent them from remembering what their destination is, what they have passed by on their way, and how to retrace their steps.

This geographic disorientation begins with an inability to find one's way when travelling outside of their hometown. They are at risk of going in the wrong direction and ending up at a completely different destination than they had intended. The area in which the person can navigate independently shrinks as their abilities decrease. Usually the next step is to lose their way when they are travelling around within their own community. People with dementia may go down a street that they have known for fifty years, and suddenly, none of the buildings look familiar. Diana Friel McGowin describes these episodes in her book, "Living in the Labyrinth," a first hand account of having dementia. They may recover their memory in a few hours, until the next episode of 'blankness', but eventually, their memory of the geography of their community is gone permanently. People who are still driving may possess driving skills, but at some time reach a point at which they are reliant on another person to be in the car with them to give them directions.

There are obvious safety concerns because of geographic disorientation. When a person with dementia has geographic disorientation and their long-term memory is on a backward trek, they may start trying to walk or drive to a home that they lived in decades ago. Since they have memory loss, they may be heading for a place in a different city or a different country without realizing it, and they become easily lost. The geographic disorientation may mean that they drive around for hours until something looks familiar and they find their way home.

Often people with dementia are no longer able to recover their bearings to find their way home. They may be unaware that they are lost and unwilling or unable to ask for help. Sometimes the help they ask for is inappropriate. One family located their mother just as she was climbing into a stranger's car. She had convinced him that she lived in another city and needed to get back there. She knew her former address and her 'Good Samaritan' was touched by her distress and willing to drive her there.

When a person with dementia goes missing, it is an extreme emergency. Search and rescue studies have indicated that people with dementia are often likely to travel in a straight line until they become stuck in something like bushes or a drainage ditch. The mortality rate is high for those not found within twenty-four hours. There is information available online about search and rescue statistics, training and planning to recover people who have become lost. (Please refer to 'www.dbs-sar.com,' and also the preplan manual for long-term care facilities, "Search is an Emergency," by the Alzheimer Society of Canada, referenced in the section entitled "Suggested Reading, References and Resources"). It is important for local police to be trained in the characteristics of people with dementia who become lost so that they are able to appreciate the urgency and the need to mount an expert search quickly. One police officer, who had attended this type of training, was off-duty and relaxing in a Tim Hortons coffee shop. He recognized the confused behaviour of a gentleman with dementia and also recognized the Alzheimer Wandering Registry bracelet on his arm. After he asked the gentleman to see his bracelet, he was able to call the police dispatcher, who looked up the registration number to find his name and address. The officer was able to notify the retirement home where he lived that he had been found. In another instance, patrons of a restaurant recognized that an elderly confused person walking to a remote restaurant on an cold snowy night was unusual, and stayed with him until help came. As it turned out, he had walked over thirty miles from a nearby town trying to get to his home. The 'Grey Alert' now available in many areas is a positive step toward making the public aware of the hazardous situation of a person with dementia becoming lost.

One fellow with early stage dementia walked for nine hours. He wanted to visit his brother who lived out of town. He was not able to recall that his wife had taken him to visit his brother just the day before. Television and radio appeals by the police resulted in two people calling to say they had seen him. The local police had been trained in the patterns of wandering of people with dementia. They drove in a straight line from these two sightings and found him over fifteen miles from home. He was glad to get a ride home, but had no idea that he was lost or how long he had been walking.

It is a good idea to take safety precautions against wandering as soon as a diagnosis is received. Having the person carry a cell phone means police can locate the person as long as they are in cell phone range (by 'pinging' the GPS (global positioning system) locator in the cell phone). This requires that another person is responsible for remembering to recharge the phone and for making sure that the person takes the phone with them and that it is turned on. A personal locator, such as that provided by the company, Eyez-On, for example, allows tracking, so that even if the person with dementia has gone out of cell phone range, their last known location before they were out of range is known (www.eyez-on.com).

Some people feel that using GPS devices is unethical because this technology could be used to prevent a person from having freedom of movement. Having personally seen the anguish of a person whose family member with dementia disappeared years before and was never found, as well as knowing about many other tragic incidents, I feel their use should be encouraged. However, it is important to be mindful of a person's freedom. GPS devices should be employed only to return people who have gone missing. An example of unethical use would be to use the device to track whether they have visited with a relative that you don't want them to see and then scold them or try to prevent the visits. If they intend to visit someone and then do so, they are not lost. Having dementia does not mean that you should be prevented from exercising your free will if you are not harming yourself or others, and are not being harmed. Many of these situations are unique and difficult. Talking them over with a professional trained in counselling people to cope with dementia can be very helpful.

Since people with dementia usually have well-ingrained habits of carrying their purses or wallets, it is a good idea to have them carry family contact information even before they are at risk for being lost. Registering with a wandering registry (for example, www.safelyhome.ca) is also advisable as soon as a diagnosis is received. It is important to keep photographs of the individual on hand, both of the face and also full-length, in order to show body shape and posture (this will help searchers spot a person a distance away). Pictures should be updated every six months or so, because of the changes in appearance and weight which often occur with dementia.

This geographic disorientation progresses until the person with dementia is unable to find their way around their own neighbourhood, and later, unable to navigate to find rooms in their own home. One woman coped with this by putting a picture on the bathroom door, so whenever her husband said that he could not find the bathroom, she could call out, "It's the room with the picture of the hockey player on the door!" and thus avoid running upstairs herself to show him the door. The lack of understanding of where they are in space and how to navigate around objects can contribute to the person with dementia having difficulty going from one place to another inside the home. In one couple's home, there was a railing dividing the kitchen from the living room, with two steps down to the living room at the end of the railing, and there was a staircase to the upstairs immediately beside those steps. The carer described how she had to repeatedly coach her husband to walk beside the railing in the kitchen area to get to the steps. He usually tried to climb over the railing to go directly to where he could see her sitting in the living room. Often, when he got to the end of the railing, he would forget where he was going and he would start to climb up the staircase on the wrong side of its railing, instead of continuing down to the living room. She often had to go and lead him into the living room as a result.

People whose geographic disorientation has extended to the point that they are not able to find their way around their own home cannot be left alone, for fear that they may inadvertently walk out the door to the outside while trying to find the way to the bathroom, for example. In one instance, a fellow went out the back door of his house in February, with no coat or boots, because he thought it was the way to the bathroom. Even when he was outside, he could not rationally connect the facts that he was standing in snow, and he was outside, and feeling cold, with the fact that the bathroom couldn't possibly be there. Of course, he may have grown up using an outhouse, and fully expected the bathroom to be in the back yard. An inexpensive solution is to put a device on the door that will ring whenever the door to the outside is opened. If you live in an apartment building, you could have it installed so the device sounds in the living room or your bedroom, so it won't disturb people in nearby apartments. You may sleep better, knowing that the alarm will sound as soon as your family member has gone outside. Another solution may be to put a sign on the door that says "Outside," if they are able to read it and recognize that's not the door for which they are looking. Very often, there are stories in the newspaper of people with dementia who have not survived when they have wandered outside, and were unable to find their way back inside, especially in very hot or very cold weather.

At other times, people who leave their home are not merely opening the wrong door, but are seeking to leave home to fulfill a need, such as going to work, having forgotten that they are retired, or going 'home' to find the family they are unable to locate. Many people who do not recognize their home are restless to 'stop visiting' and return 'home.' They may be concerned about who is paying the bill for them to stay in "this place." Reassurance given in a way that does not contradict their current view of their reality is difficult to give. Being positive and confident, rather than anxious, helps when reassurance is being given. Trying to find ways to help them meet their emotional need to be useful, to be productive or to have the feeling that they are in a place where they belong may decrease the risk that they will wander. If you can figure out what the need is that they are trying to satisfy, alter whatever is triggering that need, and provide an environment of emotional reassurance and safety, you will be doing your best to prevent a wandering incident. Such an incident may happen, despite your best efforts. The alternative of having people live in locked areas means that they would have a greatly diminished quality of life. In fact, the practice of locking people up because they have a disease, in the same way someone would be imprisoned if they are convicted and sentenced for a criminal offence, may not be valid. People with dementia necessarily live in a state of risk, and sometimes their carers cannot prevent the accidents that result, no matter how great their efforts.

2.F. Sensory Changes

Four types of changes affect a person with dementia's altered perception of the environment through their senses: their vision, hearing, smell, taste, touch, and temperature and position sense. These changes are: the ability to use the senses; the access to the long-term memories to understand the meaning of what is sensed; the slowness of information processing; and, the interpretation by the brain of what the senses perceive.

The first reason that people with dementia may have an altered perception of the environment is that their senses may no longer be functioning normally. There are changes in the sense of vision. Visual acuity is worsened, and this can hasten the loss of ability to read or tell time or recognize people or things. People whose visual acuity is affected may enjoy reading large print books and later in the disease may still be able to read headline-sized print. It is important to try, as signs may help them find a familiar place in their otherwise confusing environment. Each individual is unique in their ability to use signs. In one instance, I made a sign for an elderly gentleman who repeatedly forgot that his wife took an afternoon nap every day. It said, "I am sleeping." He had started to go out the front door and down the street using his walker to try to find her every afternoon. Since he was also legally blind, the sign was made with thick black letters that were about eight inches high, on white paper and then laminated. Whenever she went for a nap, she placed it where he would see it before he went out the front door. He immediately stopped leaving the house when she was asleep.

The loss of visual depth perception, the ability to see in three dimensions, may mean that people have difficulty navigating stairs, particularly if the same colour carpet that is on the floor also goes down the staircase. Some people have had success putting a contrasting colour of duct tape along the front of each step, so the person with dementia can visualize the steps more easily. One fellow painted a contrasting stripe of colour across the edge of each step of the deck in his back yard. His family couldn't understand why he did this. He was diagnosed with dementia of the Alzheimer's type about six months later.

If a person with dementia is looking at a solid black area, or a solid white area, such as a bathtub, they may perceive a yawning bottomless hole. Putting a pastel-coloured bath mat down may increase the likelihood that they would be willing to step into the tub. Putting a drop or a few drops of blue food colouring into the water may allow them to see what they are stepping into as well. Generally, with altered depth perception, it becomes challenging to judge how high, deep, long, wide, near or far things are.

People with altered depth perception also have difficulty knowing how close they are to objects in the environment. They are therefore more likely to bump into walls and chairs, or have difficulty using escalators, or pouring liquids, or reaching out to grasp something. One fellow kept trying to sit down on a chair, and would invariably miss. His wife watched him put two chairs side by side, back up carefully, and he still ended up sitting on the floor between the chairs. She finally arranged to have a bench for him on one side of the table. People with dementia favour wide chairs or couches because their procedural memory tells them that they always sit more successfully in wider chairs. They lack a cognitive map of where they are in space in relation to the chair. You will often see someone with dementia trying to sit on a chair, only to end up on its arm or on the edge, and then slide themselves into the middle. This is an indicator that they are starting to have trouble in this area. Procedural memory training may be used to help people with dementia remember to feel the front of the chair on the back of their legs before they sit down.

Using contrasting colours can help the person with dementia distinguish items on the table. For instance, a woman who was repeatedly knocking over her glass at the table was able to do better with a brightly coloured glass that stood out against the white placemat. People with dementia may have some changes in their colour vision; however, contrasting colours can still help them navigate through their daily tasks because of the variations in lightness and darkness. If, for example, you put a meal of white cauliflower, white mashed potatoes and white chicken on a white plate, there may not be enough variation in hue, tone and shading to allow the person with dementia to distinguish the food from the plate, and the different types of food from each other.

A glare from sunlight on a shiny floor may appear to be water on the floor or to be a hole in the floor to the person with dementia. We use our logic and memory to know that the floor is continuous, and we automatically recognize the glare as being from the sunlight. A person with dementia is no longer able to use these facts and their memories to know that it is safe to walk on the area of the floor that has the glare. Stopping to see the environment through their eyes may help you identify such problems.

Peripheral vision is also decreased, and results in the development of tunnel vision. This causes people with dementia to have problems going through the environment physically. Safety is an important consideration after tunnel vision has developed. People are more likely to trip on curbs or scatter mats, which are on the ground or floor at their feet, as these are no longer in their peripheral vision. The short-term memory, which the rest of us use to remember that there is a curb coming up, even if we are not looking at it, may not assist the person with dementia to remember to take a step up at the right time.

It may easily startle a person with dementia when moving people and objects pass through their visual field from side to side, as happens when a car goes by on the road. We see the car coming 'out of the corner of our eye,' so we have warning, whereas the person with tunnel vision will not see the car until it is directly in front. Also, they may not connect the sounds they hear with the fact that a car is driving nearby. Similarly, we can connect the fact that there are sounds of a person who is approaching from behind, so we are not surprised when they step in front of us. However, a person with dementia may respond with a startled reaction to the sudden appearance of someone in front of them. It is a good idea for family members who are identifying this problem to start whistling, talking or singing as they approach in order to get the attention of the person with dementia to let them know that they are coming. The brain also becomes slower at processing visual information, which compounds the difficulty they have in processing changes in movement in their environment.

Many people have mentioned that the family member with dementia likes to walk directly behind them. This upset one lady as she and her husband had always gone on long walks side-by-side holding hands. This may be the easiest place for the person with dementia to keep track of their companion, if they have tunnel vision and their decreased peripheral vision does not allow them to easily see someone walking beside them. Once she understood this, this lady relaxed and stopped expecting him to be able to walk beside her as he used to. It made her sad, but it decreased her stress when she stopped trying to get him to do something that now made him uncomfortable.

The sense of smell may decrease, and the most notable effect when this occurs is a decrease in the ability to taste food. On our tongues, we taste sweetness, sourness, saltiness and bitterness. The rest of our ability to taste can be attributed to the sense of smell. One fellow who lost his sense of smell quite early in the disease, described how he had to force himself to eat, because the food he put into his mouth tasted like cardboard. This same fellow put six to eight teaspoons of sugar in his tea. He said he couldn't taste the tea or the milk, but he enjoyed the sensation of having hot, sweet liquids. He also enjoyed salty foods and meals that were highly spiced.

The second reason a person with dementia may have an altered perception of the environment is because they have lost memories of the meanings of sensations. This is another illustration of information disappearing from the long-term memory. For example, at some point we learn how different flowers smell or what burning toast smells like. We are able to sniff the air and think, "Those lilac flowers smell wonderful," or "Something's burning!" We learned those meanings in the past and they will eventually be forgotten with the progression of dementia.

If, for example, the person forgets what a common sound means, such as the ringing of a telephone, they will be startled every time they hear it. Most people who hear a sound they can't identify immediately want to know what the sound was, and get up to investigate until they have solved the mystery. People with dementia may have this type of startle reaction to normal, everyday sounds. Thus, they are frequently surprised, and become anxious and in need of reassurance if they become frightened. They may not be able to communicate the source of their worry. This is often the reason that people with dementia become agitated and restless for no apparent reason. Even though you do not know the reason that they have become anxious, it is important to reassure and calm them, rather than tell them that they have no reason to be anxious. The reason is there, in their reality; it is difficult to find out what it is, and you may never figure out why, but you can still reassure them that they are safe and secure.

One fellow went to visit his mother who had early dementia due to Alzheimer's disease. She told him that she could hear animals in the walls. He listened, but heard nothing whenever she said she heard the animals. After an hour or two, he realized that she said she was hearing animals each time the fan on the furnace started up. She had forgotten what the meaning of that sound was and in trying to figure it out, came to the wrong conclusion. A person with dementia who is having this type of experience may be helped by having a sign which says something like "When the furnace fan comes on, it sounds like there are animals in the wall. There are no animals in the house." A carer would have to discuss with the person with dementia whether or not they'd like a sign, what is the most helpful thing to write on the sign, whether the letters are big enough to read, and then put it where it can be easily seen, for example on the wall near their favourite chair or beside the television. This would help to calm them down when there is no one at home to reassure them.

Television or radio programs are one example of sounds and visual effects, which may disturb a person with dementia, who no longer knows the meaning attached to these media. If you can put yourselves into the mind of someone who has forgotten what a radio or television is, you may have a reaction that is not unlike someone from the 1700's, before televisions were invented, suddenly experiencing a television. You may think that the people in the box are looking at you or talking to you, or laughing at you. Unlike the person from the 1700's, if you have dementia, you will not be able to learn what that box is and become accommodated to it, because your short-term memory loss will prevent you from laying down this new permanent memory. People with dementia frequently respond to what is being said on the radio or television as if there is a real person there speaking to them.

Some people with dementia are no longer able to interpret music as sounding musical. One lady said that she could no longer listen to any music. Her brain had somehow lost the capacity to integrate the sounds into anything pleasant, and all music sounded like annoying meaningless noise to her. She was still capable of verbally stating her preferences and insisting that others should turn off any music she could hear. People with dementia may not respond when spoken to, or when there is a noise to which they should respond. It can be difficult to distinguish whether a person with dementia is having physical changes that cause deafness, or if they are not responding to the things they hear because they no longer understand what those sounds mean. This has safety considerations when it comes to being sure that the person can interpret the sound of a smoke alarm or a car honking. Helping the person with dementia to develop a new procedural memory (perhaps by using the spaced retrieval method mentioned in the section entitled "Procedural Memory") to re-establish an appropriate response to a smoke alarm may increase the safety of a person who lives alone.

People who can no longer understand what it means when they are experiencing pain need extra support for their comfort and safety. One daughter had her mother on a camping trip. The mosquitoes were biting, and everyone else at the cottage had on long sleeves and was putting on bug spray; everyone except the lady with dementia. Her daughter asked if she needed a jacket, and she refused. Later that night, her daughter felt terrible when she discovered that her mother's skin was absolutely covered in mosquito bites under her clothing. Her mother did not realize anything was wrong. Very often, this is the way carers discover that the person with dementia has had a progression in their disease process and has lost some ability. They feel very guilty when something goes wrong, but there was no possibility that they could have anticipated such a change.

Losing the ability to understand why pain is being felt and react appropriately can also lead to difficult situations. One lady had heated up a hot pack in the microwave for her husband's lower back for years at the same time every day. One day she removed it after the usual twenty minutes, only to discover that her husband's back was covered in blisters from being burned by the hot pack. Perhaps she heated it twice in the microwave; she could not remember that she had done anything differently. However she was very shocked that he hadn't removed it or said, "That's too hot." Knowing how he had failed to react made her very cautious in the future when giving him hot drinks, or setting the temperature of his bath. She felt terrible about the incident, but had no way of knowing beforehand that this would happen. I have heard a myth that "people with dementia do not feel pain." Likely it was started by a few incidents like this one. As with everything else, this is very individual. Even if the person does not express that they are feeling pain, they may still have the pain, and they certainly can be injured by something that would injure the rest of us.

There is a sense called proprioception, which we use to know the position of our body and its parts. There are baroreceptors in our body and limbs that send information to our brain so we know whether we are standing or lying down, whether our arms are at our side or we are holding them up in the air, or whether our legs are on the bed or hanging down the side of the bed. Our brains accumulate the knowledge that makes them able to interpret this information when we are growing from infancy to childhood. When this information is being lost during the progression of dementia, people have great difficulty understanding what position they are in. A carer may ask a person to lift their legs onto the bed and become frustrated when they don't cooperate. Later that day, they may lift their legs onto the bed on their own. The next time they are asked to do it, they may look puzzled and not move their legs. Even when you start to lift their legs for them, they may not understand what is happening and fail to help. The carer knows that they are able to do it, but they just don't when they are requested to do so. Sometimes the person with dementia, if they are still able to communicate verbally, will argue that their legs are already on the bed, when they clearly aren't. Rather than argue, it is better to distract them briefly and then try a different approach to help them position themselves in the bed.

People with dementia may also not be able to identify objects by touching them. Sometimes one of the items on a test to diagnose dementia is putting a small object, such as a coin or a key in their hand when their eyes are closed, to see whether they can identify it by touch. Translating what they feel in their hand into an identification of the object they are holding may no longer be possible. In addition, some people with dementia have noticed that they have numbness or an inability to feel with their fingertips, which makes identification of objects difficult.

When we are in our childhood, we also learn what various body sensations mean. We learn to identify pain and locate where we are feeling it. We learn to identify hunger, thirst and fatigue and what to do to remedy those unpleasant situations. Like other learned information, the meaning of these sensations can also be lost as the long-term memory deteriorates. One lady whose mother lived with her had to rush her to hospital when she became ill. She was very upset when she discovered that her mother had become dehydrated under her care. She didn't realize that her mother had lost the ability to interpret a feeling of thirst, and even though she was capable of going to get a glass of water for herself and drinking it, she failed to do so. She remedied the situation at home by having a special pitcher for water in the fridge for her mother. The new procedure became that her mother had to finish drinking a full pitcher of water every day.

When people with dementia feel pain, they may not remember what it is, what is causing it, and how to help themselves feel better. This can cause a great deal of agitation in the person with dementia. It is important to be certain that they are receiving pain medication if they regularly used it prior to the onset of their dementia, because of arthritis or some other painful condition. If they are unable to state that they have pain, watching their body language can be useful. Rubbing or holding their head may indicate a headache. Rubbing a joint, or groaning when they get up may indicate stiffness and pain. Walking bent over, if it is unusual for them, may mean they have a stomach ache or a full bladder. Being unwilling to move may also indicate pain.

The third thing that alters the perception of the environment is that the processing of all information by the brain slows down with dementia. This is particularly noticeable when people are receiving sensory information and then having to react to it. For example, the processing of auditory information, things that are heard, is slowed. It is helpful, when speaking to someone with dementia, to slow your speech down so they have more time to process the sounds you are making when you speak. One fellow described his initial experiences talking with a group of his friends when his dementia was just starting. He was processing the words they said slowly. Because they were speaking too quickly for him, he missed the last part of each person's contribution to the conversation. He was also slow in responding. When he did say something, his friends would look at him with shock and say, "Where have you been? We were talking about that five minutes ago!" He still had an emotional memory of these type of events months later when he related the story, and also said that he no longer did any talking when he was with his friends, he just listened to them. He was too afraid of being embarrassed.

A conversation I had with one couple illustrated the slowness of sensory information processing quite clearly. The fellow with dementia had asked me to explain short-term memory difficulties to his wife as she was continually becoming annoyed when he forgot events and conversations during the day. Usually I was in the habit of automatically slowing down when I spoke to a person with dementia, but because I was speaking to his wife, by mistake I sped up to a normal conversational pace. I stopped after I had finished saying a few sentences to her. Her husband looked at me and asked, "Were you speaking that whole time? At the beginning I heard your words, but in the middle I couldn't hear any sound, I could only see your lips moving. At the end I heard what you were saying again." His brain was processing sound so slowly that in the middle, he was still processing the sounds I had made at the beginning, so he didn't hear the sounds of the words in the middle. When I stopped at the end and there was silence, he was able to process those words. However, his visual processing was not slowed down, so he was able to see my lips move from the beginning to the end.

The fourth change that alters the ability of the person with dementia to interpret the environment around them is the brain's ability to interpret what it sensed. We are entirely dependent on our brains to tell us correctly what is in our environment, what we are sensing that is external to us, and what we are sensing about our own bodies. We expect that other people will experience what we see, hear, smell, taste and touch in the same way we do. However, when a person has dementia, their brain does not always give them accurate information.

I asked one woman what had been the first symptom of her dementia. She told me that the first thing that she could remember about the changes that she was experiencing was that she would see multiple copies of her field of vision. She compared it to the way a fly is reported to see, as if there were dozens of television screens packed together all showing the same room she was looking at.

Another lady told me about an incident with her mother who had dementia. They were out in the front yard doing some gardening. There was a young tree that had been recently planted which was about the same height as her mother. She noticed her mother seemingly talking to herself, but then when she looked more closely, her mother was talking to the tree. Then her mother turned around and said, "Come over here, this lady would like to meet you." She discovered that her mother was seeing a lady with a green dress when she looked at the tree. This is an example of the brain misinterpreting visual information.

A woman who had been recently diagnosed with dementia of the Alzheimer's type and had also had hip surgery was rehabilitating her hip by going up and down the stairs of her apartment building. However, her brain gave her misinformation about what she was doing. She said, "When I'm going upstairs, I know I am going upstairs, I can see the stairs going up, but my body is telling me that I am going down; and, when I am going downstairs, I can see I'm going down, but my body feels like it's going up." This is an example of the brain misinterpreting proprioceptive sensory information.

We sometimes refer to the misinterpretation of the environment as an illusion, and this will be further discussed in the section entitled "Delusions, Illusions and Hallucinations."

Listening closely to the person with dementia will help you understand how they perceive the environment at any one time. Stopping to recognize all the sights and sounds around you, that you are ignoring, may help you to identify something in the environment that could worry a person who doesn't understand what it means. Whenever you notice a change in the way a person with dementia is behaving or interacting with the environment, it is a good idea to carefully observe and evaluate the situation. It is quite likely that their abilities have changed. Your first indication that this has happened will be your own reaction to their behaviour: you may think to yourself, "Now, that was strange" or something similar. Your own mind is telling you that something has happened that you have never seen before. Thoughtfully puzzling about the situation and talking with the person with dementia and others will help you stay current with the changing needs for help from you that the person with dementia requires, which will decrease the stress for both you and the person with dementia.

2.G. Language and Communication

Language difficulties take many forms. Aphasia means the loss of language, and can include both speech, or expressive language, and comprehension, or receptive language. Usually, this happens gradually as the dementia progresses. Any one, or all, of these skills may be affected: understanding what others are saying; knowing what things are called; being able to think of words; and, being able to use words to communicate what you want to say. Change in the ability to physically move the muscles of the face, mouth and throat can also change the ability to express oneself with language.

The dementia caused by disease robs people of their vocabulary and their grammar. All of us are occasionally annoyed when we grope for the right word. However, when language begins to be affected by dementia, the frustration of word-finding difficulties may happen dozens of times a day. People may use a similar word such as salt when they mean sugar, or stroller when they want to say walker. They may describe the thing that they can't name: for example, a cup may be described as "the thing that I drink out of."

This difficulty in naming things is compounded by the long-term memory loss of knowing what things are. A person with dementia may look at a fork, turn it over, put it down, and be puzzled, not knowing what it is or how one would use it. The knowledge that they developed in childhood, about forks or other eating utensils, and their use, has disappeared. The loss of the ability to interpret perceptions combines with the loss of language to make communication and understanding more and more difficult. So if someone says, "Please pick up your fork;" the person with dementia may not recognize the word or the object.

The people close to the person with dementia often correct mistakes in language. This frequently provides a source of irritation or tension between them. All of us are somewhat offended anytime that people tell us that we are wrong. We might think to ourselves: "Who does she think she is, trying to tell me that I'm wrong?" It is an irritation that we have to make an effort to get over. Pointing out that someone is wrong is not something the rest of us do lightly. People with dementia make very frequent mistakes; as time goes on, they are almost always wrong. Having mistakes pointed out to them every time they are wrong causes a lot of stress, and their stress builds each time they are corrected.

Continuous patterns of negative and scolding interaction may lead to anger or withdrawal on the part of the person with the disease. Long-time carers often talk about how they learned to "just let things go," rather than correcting every mistake. When any person corrects someone else's mistake, they expect that they will learn from that correction and not make that mistake again. When a person has dementia, they are unable to learn how to do things correctly again. Learning to "let it go" is difficult, but greatly decreases the stress and frustration for both the person with dementia and the carer.

People with dementia who are having language difficulties sometimes appear to completely ignore what you are saying, as though they didn't hear it. If you think of the sounds that come out of your mouth as just that, sounds, you can realize that the person to whom you are speaking is using their brain to organize those sounds into words, and to give those words meaning, in order to understand what you are saying. Further, their brain is integrating the meaning of your communication with the other things they know in order to evaluate your words. When someone cannot sort the sounds into meanings, your words become meaningless, as though they were listening to a language being spoken that they do not understand. One fellow described his experience with this by saying, "It's not just that I need a hearing aid: I need a descrambler!"

Many people with dementia have difficulty with being asked questions. They are busy trying to understand what is being asked, and also worrying that they won't find the right words to answer, or that they won't know the answer. Carers can often find ways to get the information they need by some other means than a direct question. For example, "I guess we could go for a walk now" might be better received than "What do you want to do right now?" If they refuse the walk and suggest something else, you still have the information you needed. Canadians would probably say, "I guess we could go for a walk now, eh?" which is halfway between a suggestion and a question and implies that either acceptance or rejection of the suggestion is alright.

The problem of comprehending what others have said is made worse when the person with dementia is in a room with many people talking at once. People who do not have dementia can be in a crowded room with dozens of conversations going on at once, and they are able to selectively pay attention to only the conversation they are having, and ignore all the rest. However, in the same situation, people with dementia and language impairment, at some point during the progression of their dementia, become unable to isolate their own conversation, and instead, hear all the words in the room as a great tangled 'word salad.' Families may see the frustration this causes the person with dementia, as their loved one retires to a room alone during a family gathering; as they leave their place of worship to sit in the car to avoid all the chit chat after the service; or, when they refuse to go to restaurants or malls where there is so much to see and hear that they are totally overwhelmed and perhaps frightened. They are not able to comprehend any meaning and either stay quiet and emotionally withdraw, or try to physically leave the room because they are emotionally overwhelmed by this confusing situation. One lady in the very early part of the disease described being overwhelmed when in situations where many things are going on at once. She said she felt very insecure and anxious if she were anywhere in town besides her own home. People with dementia who are unable to selectively pay attention are best able to communicate when they are in a conversation with just one other person, they are face to face, and the other person is speaking slowly, using simple words and phrases.

When I stopped by to visit a couple in their home one day, they left the television on in the living room as we chatted in the kitchen. Every few minutes the woman with dementia would poke her husband's arm and say, "Help that lady! Why don't you help that lady?" Neither her husband nor I could figure out what she was talking about. Finally we realized that in the television program that could be faintly heard in the living room, a woman was screaming frequently. Her husband and I were able to filter out the sound from the television as inconsequential, and therefore we weren't conscious of the screams or even that the television was still on. However, the woman with dementia had lost the ability to tell whether the screams on the television were real or not, and had also lost the ability to selectively pay attention to only our conversation and ignore the background noise. When her husband got up and turned off the television, she was more able to participate in our conversation.

Many people will try to "fill in" a word or a phrase when a person with language difficulties is stuck for a word. During many discussions with people with dementia the overall feeling was that they did not enjoy this. They often just needed a little more time to find the word themselves. If they were given a word that was not the one they wanted, it was distracting and often made them forget what they were in the middle of saying. Asking people with dementia what they prefer, will give rise to different answers. Some people said they would like a suggestion for the word they are trying to find; others said they do not want suggestions; others said to wait until they ask for help; and, still others said to wait until they had tried for a little while, and then offer. Some people said that for them, it depended on who was offering! All of the people with dementia appreciated being asked what approach they preferred. They are losing control of much of their lives and acknowledging that they have control in this area is validating for them.

The carers have to become comfortable with being silent while the person tries to find the right word, because chatting while they think, will mean that they have to try to listen to you and think about their own word search at the same time. This is multitasking, or trying to do two things at once, which becomes impossible with short-term memory loss.

As mentioned briefly in the section on short-term memory loss, one thing that worked very well, mainly for people in the early stage, was giving people with short-term memory loss permission to interrupt a discussion. This was done because of so many people with dementia saying that they would think of something they wanted to say, but by the time they politely waited for a pause in the conversation, they had forgotten what it was. Interrupting became a comfortable procedure. After a person interrupted, and said what they wanted to talk about, the discussion would be facilitated by going back to the previous topic. Once the discussion was finished, the person who had interrupted would be reminded about what they had said they wanted to tell. It was rewarding to see the beaming smiles that often came back as they accepted this help to participate in a social conversation. At this early stage, having been reminded about the topic they had wanted to talk about during the conversation, they were able to successfully say what was on their mind.

People with dementia and their families were encouraged to use this strategy at home. It decreases everyone's frustration and increases communication in the family. Sometimes, when dealing with dementia, it is important to throw out the rules and create some new rules for the new circumstances. There are some carers who are very rigid in their thinking and refuse to change their expectations for polite conversation, but most are flexible and pleased to have a way to communicate more effectively.

The pattern of long-term memory loss, in which the memories that are made in the most recent years disappear first, has a bearing on language skills. If a person is able to speak two or more languages, the language learned more recently starts to disappear first. The person's first language or 'mother tongue,' which they learned as a very young child, will be available to them for the longest time. If some of the family are not able to speak that language, it is very helpful if they learn even a little of it. Being able to say simple things like "Here is a drink of juice," or "I love you," in a language the person with dementia still understands, can make an enormous difference for both the person with dementia and the carer.

Eventually, if the person with dementia lives until the late stages of their disease, they are very likely to lose all of their language function. Some people develop language changes early in their illness; others maintain their fluency for years. This does not mean that a carer should stop talking to a person who has lost their ability to understand. Explaining verbally and by showing with your hands, what you are going to do, will help the person with dementia remain calm as you help them with their daily care. Hearing your voice, if you maintain a calming and reassuring tone, will also help them to feel safe and secure.

It is important to remember that when a person with dementia hears you talk to someone else on the phone or in person, they will also react to the tone you use with another person. They are unable to differentiate what message you are aiming at them and what is meant for someone else. If you are speaking sadly or angrily to someone else, the person with dementia usually feels that your anger or discontent is aimed at them. This can cause severe anxiety and irritation.

There is a type of dementia in which the loss of language skill is the first symptom of the dementia. This is known as 'Primary Progressive Aphasia.' In most other cases of dementia, whether it is the Alzheimer type or any other, people start to have some difficulty with word-finding in the early stage of the disease, but continue to be able to use language to some extent until the later stages.

It often happens that people who have receptive aphasia are still able to express themselves, or those with expressive aphasia are still able to understand what is said. So, it is possible for people who are able to speak, to be unable to comprehend what others are saying back to them. The opposite is true as well: it is possible for people who are not able to speak at all to understand completely what another person is saying to them.

One lady, whose husband was not able to speak, was uncertain whether he could understand what anyone else said. At one point in our conversation, she mentioned some of his visitors who could always make him laugh. When I asked what they did to make him laugh, she replied that they told him stories about funny everyday events. From that, we were able to realize that he could understand what was being said: he still had his receptive language skills. This changed their time together as she was now able to read to him (slowly) and know that when she spoke, he understood. This was particularly meaningful to this couple, because she was often reading the poetry to him that he had written himself. Afterwards, he may not have remembered what she had read, but at the moment she was reading it, he would have been able to understand and enjoy it. He would then build a procedural memory of being cared about.

Early in my career, I had a personal experience, which emphasized the need to try to communicate with a person with dementia. A fellow was being transferred from a hospital to a nursing home. I asked his wife if she had told him, and she couldn't bear to do it. Whenever he spoke, it was in gibberish: few words could be understood, and he was constantly muttering to himself. I explained to him that his wife could no longer look after him at home and that he was going to the nursing home the next day. He stopped his constant pacing and stood, looking at me closely. With great effort, he said, "money money money money money." I realized that he was quite likely worrying that his wife might not be able to afford it, and indeed, it had been a struggle to help her figure out the options. I reassured him with simple words that we had found a way that she could pay for his care and still stay at their home. He nodded abruptly as if to indicate he was thinking "Good!" and was more relaxed.

Reading is also affected by decreased language skills. People who are losing their vocabulary may show frustration at no longer recognizing many words. However, it is important to remember that every person is unique. Some people are able to continue reading if the print is large, or if the passages are short, such as with poetry or simple signs of one or a few words. Other people can read flawlessly out loud, but do not understand the meaning of what they have read.

On one occasion, a sign with a person's name on his door failed to allow him to find his room in the facility in which he was receiving care. This fellow was perfectly fluent in speaking English. However, further observation revealed that the books he was reading were in Persian, and this led to the realization that the sign also needed to be written in Persian. The family's help in making this happen resulted in his ability to be successful in finding his room. Another lady was able to easily read the sign with her name on it, but she also did not use it to find her room in the long-term care home. Watching her as she walked down the hall and thinking about what she was looking at, provided the solution. Her back was permanently bent, so that when she was walking, she would have been able to see only the bottom eighteen inches of the door. The sign had been placed at everyone else's eye level. Moving it down the door to where she could see it, allowed her to make use of this valuable environmental cue. Very often, when dealing with dementia, one is reminded of the saying to "Think outside the box." On many occasions, you find yourself thinking: "Box? What box?" Sometimes the problem is so unusual, you feel like there is no standard "box." Creative thought is very helpful, and many minds working together are even more helpful.

It often happens that people with dementia who have decreased language skills say unexpected things that we find very funny. Some people have mixed feelings about whether or not they should laugh. Many people with dementia enjoy the fact that they have created laughter, even though they find it difficult to understand exactly what was so funny. This is a long, difficult and sad disease. If you can find things to laugh about, by all means enjoy them. It is important for the person with dementia to feel that they are not being laughed at, rather, that you are laughing with them. Giving them a big hug and telling them they are wonderful will get this message across. Be careful to watch their expressions if you tell the story in front of them. Be thoughtful and sensitive to their feelings. If it makes them proud and happy, by all means continue. If they look embarrassed and leave the room, it is better to stop. Shared laughter is a treasure. As one carer said to me, "You have to laugh. If you don't laugh, you cry. Lots of times you laugh and cry at the same time."

It is important to remember when you are caring for someone with dementia, as was mentioned in the section on emotions, that spoken language is not the only way to communicate. Our body language, our smiles, relaxed posture, warmth in the tone of voice we use, playing a game such as tapping each other, a fond touch, holding hands, or stroking an arm, communicate our feelings and the idea that the person is important to us. Since a person with dementia may not recognize what role an individual is playing in their lives, all carers of the person with dementia, whether they are family or not, should communicate their positive feelings in these non-verbal ways, if they are well-received by the person with dementia.

In some instances, communication of your intentions by using only body language works better than speaking words. If you say to a person with dementia, "Come and walk with me in the yard," they have to process your words to figure out what you want and then figure out how to answer, as well as what actions they should perform next. Often, when people with dementia cannot figure out what you are saying, they just respond with "No." If instead, you face the yard, smile and hold out your hand to take their hand, it expresses the same information more simply.

As people with dementia begin to lose their language skills we need to accommodate to the changes they are experiencing that affect their ability to communicate: memory loss; language loss; a decreased ability to process information; and a lack of ability to control their expression of emotions. Communication with a person who has no dementia is a shared responsibility. When one person has dementia, the well person shoulders all the responsibility for the way the conversation goes. For example, if a person with dementia is telling a story we know is not true, rather than upset them by arguing, it may be better to just listen. Being contradicted, argued with, or being accused of lying can cause great upset to the person with dementia. Their brains may no longer be able to discern fact from fiction at times. It will create great stress for the person with dementia if someone wants to "test" their memory by constantly asking if they remember this or that. It is important to avoid being judgemental, scolding, correcting, exasperated, and impatient, or treating them like a child. Exhibiting our impatience and frustration and forcing the person with dementia to cope with it, can cause them to respond in ways that they no longer understand are uncivil; and they cannot prevent themselves from responding in these ways. Using a respectful tone of voice, listening to them with interest and accepting them as they are, helps both the person with dementia as well as the carer. Supporting the person with dementia means not creating situations where the frustration becomes overwhelming for them. Trying to have an approach to the person with dementia of unconditional positive regard helps carers judge their actions. This means that whatever the person with dementia does or says, they are treated in a kindly and positive manner.

Often in the early stage, when people with dementia are relaxed, they go from point to point in a conversation with very little repetition. The conversation does, however, take unexpected turns and flights to different topics, rather than one point logically progressing from the other. However, that can be quite interesting. These are people with a lifetime of experience and wisdom to share, and it helps if we accept the way they are able to communicate it.

Also in the early stage, people with dementia may choose to talk about difficult life and death issues. It is important to maintain the person's topic of conversation, without switching it to something with which you are more comfortable. In order to communicate with them, we need to deal with our own grief, and acknowledge to ourselves why we are feeling uncomfortable, before we can meet their need to converse about their dilemmas, sad thoughts, and concerns. The conversation will then be more meaningful to both. For example, if someone talks of death, it is important to let them talk, rather than dismiss their need by saying something like, "No, we don't want to hear that kind of talk around here!" In these situations, it's not so important what you say in return. What is important is how intently and respectfully you listen.

Increasing the meaningful communication in the family is important. Many families have regular meetings; about every six months is average. At times, family members will talk about some aspect of caring that they have trouble with and find that others have worked out a solution. Once you find out what works well for the person with dementia, don't keep it a secret! Staying connected and supportive to each other helps everyone.

2.H. Time Disorientation

The person with dementia loses the ability to use time in a meaningful way fairly early in the illness. This includes the ability to know the meaning of what time it is, what time of day it is, what day of the week it is, the month, the season, or the year.

People with dementia, who wear a watch and are able to read it, will often check their watches very frequently. They are not able to hold the information about what time of day it is in their short-term memory, after thinking about or talking about something else distracts them. When a person is well, frequent checking of their watch when they are engaged in conversation is taken as meaning they are bored and anxious to get away, and the others they are with may feel a bit insulted. So, it is very important not to take the frequency of time checking by a person with dementia as a personal insult.

Before the onset of dementia, most people have developed a good sense of how much time has elapsed since they last checked the time. Since the person with dementia has difficulty remembering what time it was when they last checked their watch, they also have difficulty knowing how much time has gone by. Those people with dementia who can no longer read a watch or clock have even more difficulty telling how much time has elapsed. The person who lives with them may go out to the store for an hour, and when they come back they are greeted with "Why have you been gone so long? It's been hours!" The opposite can also happen, where hours have gone by and the person with dementia thinks that only a few minutes have passed. They may also seem quite unaware of time passing at all. This is an issue when you both have to be somewhere on time, and you feel as though you have to constantly remind them to take the next step toward getting ready to leave.

We connect many different thoughts and hold them in our memory simultaneously in order to tell what time of the day it is. We may understand that it is two o'clock in the afternoon by knowing that we finished lunch about an hour ago, or that we have been at work for five or six hours and how far we have gotten in our daily routine. If we are outdoors or we can see out a window, we know that it is daylight, and that helps us to orient ourselves. We can sense by the position of the sun and the brightness of the daylight whether it is morning, mid-day or evening.

All of these factors add together to orient us to the time of day. When a person has dementia, they are disconnected from these reminders. They may have forgotten that darkness means it is night, and that there are many activities that we usually do only in the daytime. They may go out for a walk in the middle of the night, or not understand why they cannot call a family member on the telephone at three o'clock in the morning.

In order to remember what day it is, we need to form a memory of what day it was the day before, which is not done when short-term memory loss is present. Similarly, people with dementia may be unable to remember what month it is, having never formed a memory for what the previous month was. As the long-term memories available to the individual regress back in time, they may often forget what year it is. Sometimes when you ask a person with dementia what the year is, they will very confidently state a year that is twenty years earlier or more. From this we can get a clue about where, in time, their context is at that moment.

Many families have told a story about the person with dementia practising the day, month and year all the way to the doctor's office, knowing that they are about to have this aspect of their memory assessed, only to forget it when they are asked during the assessment. This presents an interesting observation about the new procedural memory they have made: they can remember that they have this assessment and that they can never remember the date when asked. They remember the procedure, but not the date. One lady's husband, a retired medical doctor, was so upset by his repeated failures to remember the date, that she and their doctor agreed that he would never have to go through that type of assessment again. It made no difference to his treatment and he found it stressful, so they thoughtfully discontinued it.

A person may not remember having breakfast, and telling them that it is 10:30 A.M. and well past breakfast may work for a couple of minutes until their short-term memory fails, and they ask again about breakfast. They may not recognize the feeling of fullness in their stomach as indicating that they don't need to eat again, as they are no longer able to connect bodily sensations to the meaning of those sensations. Working to find out what will allow them to stop repeatedly asking for breakfast will help decrease their anxiety. The anxiety may not be about eating at all. There may be some other basis for the anxiety, but it is being expressed as a worry about when they are going to eat. Looking at their whole emotional and physical environment may be necessary before appropriate reassurance and calming can be found.

An example of time disorientation is a story about a security guard. He started work at eight in the morning; however, as his sense of time eroded with the beginnings of his Alzheimer's disease, he began to arrive at work earlier and earlier. He knew that his ability to tell time was not functioning, so he began pushing himself to get out the door as soon as possible after he woke up. The anxiety caused him to wake earlier, and after a few months he was regularly showing up for work about 4 A.M. This almost obsessive over-compensation for memory loss is not unusual amongst people with dementia.

Tasks that are repeated during the day are confused when the element of lapsed time is taken into consideration. Drying the dishes after one meal blends in with drying the dishes after every other meal. One lady asked her husband every time they did the dishes why he had made them dirty again because they had just finished them. In reality, hours had gone by between each episode of doing the dishes.

There are many safety concerns when a person is disoriented to time. The food will go bad in the refrigerator because they do not remember how many days it has been since they bought it. People will carefully take their medication, and then do it again half an hour later, forgetting they have previously taken enough for the day. People with a medication dossette will do the same, forgetting what day it is. A person who is disoriented to time may go for a walk in the middle of the night, or set out to go to work at a job they used to do decades ago, perhaps in a different city or country. Sometimes simple solutions are effective. One lady piled up three or four empty cookie tins in front of the door at night. She knew that the noise they would make when they toppled over if the outside door was opened would wake her up. When her husband asked why she was doing this, she said it was to let them know if anyone was breaking into the house, and her explanation satisfied him.

The learned ability to read a watch is eventually lost. One fellow related to me that he was able to tell the time again after he was given a watch with large numbers. Later in his dementia, he said that he could tell what hour it was, but could not differentiate partial hours, such as "a quarter to" or "twenty past." He remembered that he used to be able to do this, but no longer could, a procedural memory. Still later, he wore the watch out of habit, but no longer used it.

Some people are better able to read the time from a digital clock, than one with an analogue clock face. There are clocks that will "speak" the time when a button is pushed, and other clocks which display the day and date, as well as the time. Such devices may allow a person to reorient themselves to the time as long as they are able to do so.

There has been a debate in the past about trying to reorient people with dementia to the date. Their short-term memory loss does not allow them to remember being told the date. If they are expected to remember, they feel stress and a sense of failure when they are unable to recall the date. This may cause them to withdraw socially, and refuse to participate in activities. Trying to reorient someone to 'reality,' in general, does not help the person with dementia who cannot remember what has been said and whose own reality is altered so drastically by their disease process.

2.I. Loss of Initiative

When the part of the brain that controls initiation of activity or communication is damaged, people become less able to start an activity or a conversation. The term 'apathy' is sometimes used to describe this symptom. However, the word apathy is more suited to describe those who lack interest, curiosity, motivation and desire to participate, because of their mood, rather than those who are physically and intellectually incapable of driving their own actions to carry out an action or desire that they have conceived. People with dementia, who have this lack of ability to initiate, need to rely on other people to cue them, in order to be involved in conversation or in activities.

Families talk about their frustration because the person just sits and stares at nothing for long periods of time, and feel that they should be using their time for some purpose. When this occurs, it is important to identify who has the problem. Is the person with dementia being harmed by sitting for long periods, or is it the carer's discomfort with this change in the person's state that is the issue? The disease process causes the lack of initiative. As long as the person is receiving adequate nutrition, is getting sufficient exercise spaced throughout the day, and is sitting in a soft comfortable chair so they are not at risk to develop pressure areas, and they seem relaxed, and are not showing signs of anxiety stemming from boredom, then their condition should be accepted. Periodic stimulation and pulling them into engagement with activities and conversation are useful, however, the person will not exhibit full-time engagement with those around them and their environment as they had previously.

Many family members have said something like "I think I'd go crazy if that were me, just sitting around doing nothing." When this is the sentiment, it is likely that the carer is having the problem with the lack of activity of the person with dementia. However the person with dementia may be perfectly content at that moment. People with dementia should definitely be stimulated to participate in conversations and activities, but not every time they sit and stare, seemingly doing nothing. Trying to keep them constantly busy will result in excess stress, both for the person with dementia and their carer. Part of the reason that carers tend to prod people into staying busy is their rage against the devastation the disease is having on their loved one. To pull back and tolerate periods of inactivity means that they have to emotionally accept the disease and its relentless progression, which is very difficult for all family and friends.

2.J. Sexuality and Intimacy

In the early stage of dementia, there may be no changes in the pattern of sexual intimacy in a relationship. On a few occasions, I was asked whether sexual relations should stop, as a result of having a diagnosis of a disease causing dementia. My answer was to make the decision according to the response of the individual with dementia. If both members of the couple are willing and find sexual intimacy pleasurable and emotionally comforting, there is no reason to stop.

The changes in the long-term memory can have a great impact on sexuality. As a person's context slips back in time (if the Alzheimer pattern of retrograde amnesia is present), they may relate to sexuality as they may have as a younger person. Some men and women may develop a heightened interest in lovemaking, which their spouses were familiar with from their younger years. This can be a positive situation for their spouse who is their carer, or it can be a negative situation. On occasion I was asked if I thought an unwilling spouse should have sexual relations with their partner with dementia who desires it. My response was always no. There are many demands on a carer, but all caring should be voluntary. Forced sexual relations are not acceptable in any situation. However, many spouses continue to accept the sexual advances of their partner with dementia, not because they enjoy it, but because they want to provide that comfort. They are making a voluntary decision. The desire for sexual intimacy typically decreases as the dementia worsens. Spouses may feel some relief when the sexual demands on them are no longer present. They may also feel guilt at their relief because it comes as a result of the person's condition worsening.

It may be important to the individual with dementia to think that they are successful lovers, even though they are no longer physically capable of lovemaking. More than one spouse shared that they would keep their spouse's self-esteem intact, even though nothing had actually happened. Other spouses told how their partners with dementia seemed frightened of them once they were unable to remember them as their spouse. They slept as far away as possible on the bed, or asked their partner to sleep in another room.

The misidentification of other people by the person with dementia as a result of their long-term memory loss is a normal and expected occurrence with dementia. When misidentification occurs in the realm of sexuality it causes many serious issues. One young lady related how relieved she was to find out about the misidentification caused by long-term memory loss. She had been horrified one day when she was chatting with her beloved grandfather who had Alzheimer's disease. He had gently reached out and touched her in a sexual manner. She felt horrified and betrayed by him. After she understood the pattern of memory loss he was experiencing, she also thought about how often she'd been told she resembled her grandmother as a young woman. She was able to hold him in high esteem again after she realized that his pattern of long-term memory loss had caused him to mistake her for her grandmother, since he was thinking that his wife was a young woman.

A daughter or son may be acutely embarrassed and concerned if their parent invites them to bed. One daughter was so relieved to find out that her father was misidentifying her, that she cancelled her plans to move him into a nursing home. After that, every time he invited her to bed at night, she would laugh and say, "No Dad, you'll be sleeping alone tonight." Her horror and embarrassment disappeared once she understood the situation. She was able to return to her previous determination to keep him with her in her home, and if possible, never put him into a nursing home. There was no change in his behaviour, but there was a change in her understanding and attitude.

Adult children may be disgusted and declare that their family will no longer visit Grandma and Grandpa. In one extended family, learning about long-term memory loss and the effect it has on misidentification completely reversed this decision. The long-term memory loss of the person with dementia causes them to forget the identity of the person and their relationship. Once the family understood this, they were able to reverse their decision to have nothing to do with their elderly parents, but to continue to help with the care of the person with dementia, while at the same time making sure that the vulnerable young people in the family were not left alone with them, and were protected from psychological damage.

Gentle teasing of an older person with dementia by a younger person that they are their "boyfriend" or "girlfriend," has led to the person with dementia being totally serious about planning to marry them. The long-term memory loss leads to the person with dementia thinking they are much younger; they misunderstand the fact that they are being teased and believe the whole situation is quite real. This is a highly emotional subject and can cause much stress and humiliation to the person with dementia and their family.

People with dementia who are in long-term care settings have similar issues. Someone who has forgotten that they are married may develop a close friendship with another resident with dementia. They may spend much of their days together holding hands when they walk together, and sitting closely side-by-side. One lady talked about how her husband walked up to her, knowing that he knew her, but not who she was, and beaming, introduced her to another woman he called "my wife." She understood that it was the dementia that caused him to forget that she was his wife. However, this situation did mean that her grieving was more difficult. Some family members are determined that their parent or spouse with dementia should not form a new such friendship in the nursing home, and insist that the staff should keep them apart. This is an unreasonable expectation, since the ideal atmosphere is to let people wander in their living quarters at will, without being restricted. The family's viewpoint is certainly understandable, and is part of the reason that having a loved one with dementia in the family is so very emotionally painful. However, from the point of view of the person with dementia, they have a very pleasant companionship.

Misidentification is a normal pattern in dementia. Similar misunderstandings can occur with care workers in the home or the nursing home who are bathing and giving other intimate care to the person with dementia. If, because of their dementia, they do not understand that they are receiving help with their bathing, they may view the activities as sexual fondling. There are two realities in play. Seeing themselves as legitimate sexual partners, the person with dementia responds in kind. The staff member's reality is that they are bathing a frail elderly person with dementia and they feel violated if that person does anything that is sexually suggestive.

It may also happen that the person with dementia may view being bathed by a stranger as a sexual attack, especially if such an attack happened to them when they were younger. Care must be taken to always perform the bath in the way they tolerate the best, to maintain their privacy, and to make no movements that are anything but slow, kind and gentle. The person with dementia will relax over the months as they form a procedural memory that they are safe in this situation.

Knowing what is causing this misunderstanding is the only way to alter the circumstances. Staff members cannot be expected to tolerate unwanted sexual advances as part of their workplace environment. It may mean that the long-term care facility must specify the gender of the care worker for the personal care of a particular resident with dementia. It may mean always having two care workers bathe the individual, one to distract the individual and the other to do the bathing.

It is vital to understand that such difficult misunderstandings are a normal result of dementia. It is a situation that can lead to very emotional and angry responses, but it is important to realize that neither the person with dementia, nor their family, nor the staff member is to blame for the situation. It is a problem that should be expected and dealt with in a calm manner, in order to restore a positive and caring emotional environment for all concerned.

2.K. Catastrophic Reactions

One gentleman tried arguing with his eighty-six-year-old wife when she insisted on going home to see her parents, who had been deceased for decades. She remained insistent and started to go out the door. Since it was dark, he was very worried about her. He tried to physically hold her back from leaving. Their daughter happened to come over shortly after and found her elderly parents rolling on the floor and hitting each other. He was trying to hold onto his wife, and to prevent her from becoming lost outside on a cold dark night; his wife was determined to fend him off so she could go 'home' to visit her parents. This couple had lived happily through many decades of marriage with no violence whatsoever. The police had to be called to settle the situation and the lady received sedation in hospital. After this gentleman learned about the changes in memory processes that were affecting his wife's behaviour, this type of episode was never repeated. If she asked to go home to visit her parents, he would say "Sure!" and they would get into the car together. He would suggest stopping for tea or an ice cream cone on the way, and gradually lead the conversation into different topics. Eventually she forgot where they were going, and they would drive home again, making plans for what they would do next.

Think of the situation that you are in right now. If someone were to tell you that some element of your reality is not true, you would laugh and think they were being ridiculous. If they continued to insist on a different version of reality than you are experiencing, you may become very annoyed, and eventually very angry with them. This is similar to a person with dementia being told that they are wrong about something they feel is obviously true.

The long-established habit of trusting their memory and reasoning is automatic in people with dementia, just as it is in people without dementia. From the point of view of the person with dementia, they are faced with another person who is being unreasonable and unfair. They are not able to realize that their judgement is impaired because of their faulty memory. To the woman in the previous story, it was absolutely right for her to be a good daughter and to visit her parents. She would have seen her husband as being mean and therefore not trusted him.

Solving disputes with other people is something we learn. A child will throw a punch at their brother or sister when Mom isn't looking, or wrestle with neighbourhood friends. As the same child grows up, they learn that behaving properly toward another human being does not include hitting and punching or other physical violence. Peaceful conflict resolution, as a learned skill, may be forgotten when a person develops dementia. So when a person with dementia reacts to a situation, as they perceive it, they are working without many memories and skills that would have helped them to an appropriate judgement and response in the past.

Here is another example of a catastrophic reaction. One woman with Alzheimer's lived in a nursing home and her husband visited every day. Every day she spent most of the visit scolding him, saying that he never came to visit her. He realized that she had no memory of his daily visits and put up with the scolding with patience and good nature. However, one day another visitor yelled at her in anger, scolding her severely for being so unfairly critical of her husband. The woman with dementia physically attacked this scolding visitor. When she was scolded, the person with dementia felt threatened. Already upset and in despair by feeling abandoned, this undeserved scolding was more than she could bear. This is a clear example of how behaving thoughtfully toward a person with dementia can help them avoid catastrophic reactions.

Another fellow was in the habit of wandering in and out of other people's rooms in the nursing home. In that home, people with dementia were in the same part of the home as people without dementia. One resident who did not have dementia began to yell at him to get out of her room. Many staff members came and were talking to him all at once about leaving the room. Some were touching him, trying to physically guide him out of the room. This was an overwhelming situation for the person with dementia and he began to throw things at people and to take swings at them. Now, it is important to put yourself thoughtfully in the shoes of this man with dementia. He had no idea that he had done anything wrong, and as far as he was concerned, many people were rushing toward him to gang up and attack him. It would have been much less threatening to him if only one person had asked the other resident to stop yelling and quietly given him a big smile and held out their hand for the fellow with dementia to take and enticed him down the hall to an alternate activity.

It is important to recognize that people with dementia who are in nursing homes may have no idea where they are. This is also the first time that they have ever lived in a place where they couldn't go anywhere they wanted to in their home because they owned it. People with dementia are unable to learn how to conduct themselves appropriately. They are unable to learn how to give other residents their privacy, or to understand where the unmarked physical barriers are between the public and the private areas. This is one reason that people with dementia may be better served by being on a unit with others who also have dementia. They are all able to wander at will.

Think of how you would react if you were walking on a street and were suddenly approached by a group of people yelling and frowning at you. Would you feel threatened? Would you feel like your physical safety was at risk? Of course you would. If someone, who is yelling and frowning, reached out toward you, would you hit out to protect yourself? You have no idea why such a thing would be happening; neither does the person with dementia. They are unable to remember or reason what the context is that would give rise to what seems like a terrifying personal attack. Thoughtfulness means putting yourself in the place of the person with dementia, understanding the context, as they perceive it, and then altering your behaviour so that they no longer feel threatened. Once you understand that they are feeling threatened, increasing the physical distance between you and the person with dementia is the best way to decrease their perception of being threatened. Take a step or two back, smile, and relax.

It is the context, the meaning of the situation, which the person with dementia is not able to understand. Having context allows you to judge whether you are in danger from another person or whether they have kindly intentions toward you. Imagine you are walking through a parking lot. A stranger comes up to you, says nothing, and reaches out to touch your back. You would at least feel uncertain, if not threatened and frightened. Now suppose instead of being silent, the stranger had said, "Hold still, I'm just going to get that big spider off your back." That gives you the context; the meaning of the situation, and, you would be able to cooperate. How can we help people with dementia understand a context? We cannot give them the full context, particularly if they do not have the capacity to understand spoken language. However, we can give them a context of their own personal safety by body language signals such as remaining calm, friendly and smiling. We can decrease the noise of others shouting by asking them to stop and to leave the room. We can increase the empty physical space around them by moving away so they do not feel in imminent physical danger. This may help prevent the person from having a catastrophic reaction.

A catastrophic reaction happens when people are so overwhelmed that they react in an overtly violent manner. I do not like to use the term aggressive to describe this behaviour, because that, to me, means planning and carrying out deliberate harm to a person. Aggressive would be an apt description for someone, who has no dementia, who commits robbery or murder, for example. It is important to understand the occurrence of a catastrophic event with a person with dementia as firstly, a reaction to circumstances, and secondly, as a defensive action to protect themselves from harm when they feel threatened. Sometimes people with dementia form procedural memories of being repeatedly 'under attack.' They may strike out as soon as someone approaches them to do personal care. This may look to the carer as though they have struck out 'for no reason.' Backing away and trying another approach an hour or two later may be necessary to avoid a catastrophic reaction.

It is not an easy thing to detach yourself from the context as you know it and try to understand the viewpoint of the person with dementia. On one unit where I worked years ago, we were excited about having a new whirlpool tub for patients. We thought, "What a wonderful experience for older people with aches and pains!" To prevent staff members from injuring their backs, there was a chair with a hydraulic lift in which the patients could sit to be raised over the edge of the tub and be slowly lowered into the warm water, with it's soothing jets and bubbles. Most patients enjoyed it, however, one fellow with dementia yelled and hit and tried to bite the staff as they helped him into the tub. Puzzled, we nevertheless took this as a "no," a refusal of care, which it clearly was, and planned for a different way to help him stay clean. A few weeks later I was at home cooking and looking at the pot of water boiling on my stove. I suddenly realized that a person with dementia could view being lowered into a whirlpool tub as being lowered into a pot of boiling water. If he had never experienced a whirlpool tub before, or didn't remember them, and could not understand a verbal explanation being offered to him at the time, this could have been the context he had perceived.

Being respectful of the refusal of care of a person with dementia is important. They may not be able to say what they do not want and why, but they are definitely capable of showing it. Once a paid carer asked me about a difficult situation where she worked. There was a fellow who would start yelling with fear the moment she appeared with the shower chair. He continued to yell all the way through his shower, and stopped only when he was back in bed and the chair had been removed from the room. She asked what she should do. I said to stop showering him. There are many acceptable ways to help a person stay clean. Repeatedly forcing him through a procedure that he finds terrifying is not a kindness and not a palliative treatment for a person dying from a fatal disease.

Sometimes there are many contributing factors to a person with dementia having a catastrophic reaction. It is important to look at their physical and emotional environment and evaluate what could be causing stress. Pretend you are that person and that you know nothing about your surroundings. Is it the television show with its screams and gunfire? Remember that a person with dementia may think this is real. Is it the music on the radio that they hate? Think of a type of music that grates on your nerves, which you have to turn off instantly. Ask yourself how many hours of being forced to listen to it would it take before you felt like pitching the radio out the window? You might think your feelings are quite reasonable in the circumstances, but if a person with dementia actually did that, they might be labelled as aggressive, and given medication to sedate them, without anyone realizing that the music was the problem. Throwing the radio down may be the only way they can think of to stop the grating music. However, if the person with dementia cannot relate the source of their irritation to the radio, their agitation and frustration may cause them to strike out at something, or at someone.

Pain is one element of the physical environment that is often overlooked as a possible cause of agitation or catastrophic reactions. Two people I have known, who were in the early stage of dementia, talked about the people who came into their homes and kicked them in the knees. That was not real, but they both had arthritis in their knees. Neither one remembered that they had arthritis or what it is. They did not know why they had the pain in their knees, and they imagined, and then believed, an explanation they felt was reasonable: that they must have been kicked. If you have someone who is already living with this type of stress, feeling that they are regularly having their home invaded and their person attacked, and you add in more stressors, a catastrophic reaction is even more likely. This pattern of having the feeling first, and making up what they believe is the explanation for the feeling afterwards, can be seen in other areas of functioning by the person with dementia. If these ladies later decide who is kicking them in the knees, they may strike out at that individual. It may be that they will feel the pain when someone takes them for a walk and decide that the person who is helping them is causing the pain. Keeping careful track of such reactions may help you to understand that they are striking out whenever they have to walk. Often people with dementia are put on a trial of regular pain medication for a few weeks to see if this decreases their episodes of agitation and catastrophic reactions.

Once a person is having a catastrophic reaction it is not always necessary to forcibly remove them and restrain them. Removing others from the room and leaving them alone will allow them to calm down slowly. Although approaching in a friendly manner may be helpful in avoiding the catastrophic reaction, once they have reached that explosive emotional state, it is best to pull back and not approach in any manner, no matter how nice. Many people instinctively start to yell at the person and demand that they stop behaving badly. This will also be misunderstood, and is likely to reinforce the understanding of the person with dementia that they are being threatened and need to protect and defend themselves. Sometimes carers respond harshly because they don't want to 'indulge' or 'spoil' the person with dementia. Such a person will not 'learn' that they can 'get away with bad behaviour.' They will most often forget the incident altogether, and if the circumstances are such that they never feel threatened in the future, it may never occur again.

Sometimes there is a delay in a person's reaction. One fellow, who was a resident in a nursing home, began to hit people in a random way, that seemed to have no relationship to any context of the environment. When the events of his days were carefully tracked, it was discovered that he hit one or two people on days when he had received his morning care from a woman, but not when male staff had looked after him. Since his reaction of hitting out was twenty to thirty minutes later than the care being given, the cause of his distress was not understood at first. Once he consistently received care from a male staff member, his catastrophic reaction of hitting other people stopped.

It is important to realize that people with dementia may not remember the catastrophic reaction, but you will. You may signal that you do not trust them with your body language. Try to eliminate any outward signs of nervousness or a judgemental attitude from your approach in order to maintain their trust and to communicate that they are safe in your care.

Catastrophic reactions need to be seen as communication from a person with dementia that the situation they are in is absolutely intolerable to them. It may be the only way they have to relay this information. It is vital to figure out what is causing them to feel such distress and to change whatever it is in their physical environment, in the pattern of care they are given, or in their bodily discomfort to decrease their stress. This is emotional palliative care.

2.L. Delusions, Illusions and Hallucinations

Delusions occur when a person with dementia believes something is true, which is not actually true, based entirely on how they think about it. Illusions are the result of the brain misinterpreting something in the external environment that they have experienced through their senses. Hallucinations happen when the brain of the person with dementia creates visions, sounds, smells, tastes, or physical sensations of touch or body position which are not real.

2.L.i. Delusions

Memory loss is the main reason that people have delusions. If the person with dementia does not remember what their husband looks like or that they are married, due to long-term memory loss, they will have a delusion that the man who is in their house is not their husband. It takes a great deal of patience and learning to care for a person who does not recognize you. One elderly gentleman was able to care for his wife at home for over two years after she stopped knowing who he was. He did not press her to believe that he was her husband. He had many ways of entertaining her. She was a singer, and continued to enjoy music and singing throughout her journey with dementia. He used music repeatedly to distract her from worrying about who he was. Eventually, she had to be admitted to a nursing home because she would no longer accept his care. This was an unexpected crisis. One day she left the house and went into the street demanding that the neighbours remove "that man" from the house. Despite repeated attempts to calm her down and help her relax, she no longer felt safe.

Long-term memory loss led to one woman demanding entry to a neighbour's house to inspect it. She had the delusion that she was their landlord. After much thought, the family remembered that over forty years before in another town, the couple had owned and rented out a house across the street. Although they were upset at first, the neighbours began to invite her in if they had time for a chat, and call her husband to say she was there. He would then have to think of some reason to convince her to come back to their own home.

Having the mistaken idea that the fifty-year-old woman in front of her was a stranger, one elderly mother asked her daughter, "Who are you and what have you done with my daughter?" It was a double emotional blow for this woman's daughter. She was not recognized by her own mother and, furthermore, was also accused of being dishonest by her. When she said, "I'm your daughter!" her mother replied, "My daughter is only a little girl and you are a grown woman. You are not my daughter!" Becoming angry with the person with dementia only reinforces their mistaken belief that the person they are talking to is up to no good. It was the long-term memory loss that led to the delusion that the person in front of her was not her daughter. This elderly lady was not trying to be difficult or unpleasant. She was genuinely concerned about the welfare of her daughter. Quite likely the lady she saw as a middle-aged stranger, in front of her, reminded her of her daughter and had called her 'Mom,' which would give rise to her need to make sure her daughter was alright. This is the emotional need that needs to be met. She needs to be assisted to feel that her daughter is fine. Treating her as though she is talking nonsense will increase her anxiety, not heal the emotional symptom she is experiencing.

One woman had run a home day care for preschoolers when she was middle aged. After she developed dementia, she would start to look for the children, usually late in the afternoon when she often became agitated. The family were forced to make up the story that all the parents had come to pick up their children already. On days when she was particularly hard to calm down, her husband would take her out for a drive, pretending to look for the children in the neighbourhood. He would start chatting about different topics until she stopped worrying about the children, and then they would return home. Her emotional need to find the children was being met by having her husband believe her and take her seriously, by taking her out to look for them. That would start to decrease her anxiety. Talking about topics that were pleasant would have further calmed her anxiety, until she was calm and reassured.

There are many other examples of delusions stemming from long-term memory loss. No longer recognizing their home leads people to believe they are not at home. One woman, who also couldn't remember how much money she had, and what bank it was in, looked around her daughter's home and said, "You've done a lot of renovations to my house, and you probably used my money to do it!" In the early stage of the disease, it is often too obvious to the person with dementia for the carer to just change the topic in an effort to distract. However, a related topic may work. If this daughter had asked her mother, "Do you like the colour of the paint in the kitchen?" the conversation could move from there to some other concrete object in the kitchen, such as the stove, and from the stove to cooking. Soon, her mother would have been contentedly talking about something that did not worry her.

Constantly helping the person with dementia to focus their thoughts on topics that do not make them feel emotionally desolate is challenging and exhausting for the carer. Surfing is a good analogy. You get onto the board and up on a wave. You ride it successfully for a while. Then you fall off. Things are upset for a while. You find a new wave, get back on, and your relationship is calm again. The longer you are doing this, the better you get at knowing how to help the person with dementia become calm and you become increasingly able to prevent them from getting upset in the first place.

Many people are under the delusion that they are still working and will go to great lengths to get away from their carers to get to work. This is a safety concern. Their need to work can often be met by helping them satisfy their need to feel useful. Finding an uncomplicated one-step task and rewarding them with thanks and praise is helpful. One woman, whose husband had dementia, was absolutely determined that her husband would not 'mess up' her kitchen. She missed many opportunities to help him feel useful by perhaps peeling the potatoes, or cutting the cucumber, or any other small task. The person with dementia will usually take a long time to finish their simple task, so if you are preparing a meal, it is a good idea to let them prepare an ingredient that you won't need to use for fifteen or twenty minutes.

Thinking that their parents are alive is also a delusion. It is helpful if all the family and friends are not only aware that the person has this delusion, but are also told the best way to answer questions about the parents. These answers must be worked out by the carer through trial and error to see which response will help the person with dementia to find peace of mind.

One woman looked out the front window when her husband drove into their driveway. She could see the headrest of the empty passenger seat beside him. She had the illusion that the headrest was the head of a woman that she did not know, and this illusion gave rise to the delusion that her husband was having an affair. Her long-term memory loss would also have contributed to this illusion if her mind had the context of the way car seats looked before headrests were in common use. Having the delusion that her spouse is with another woman does not indicate that sometime in the past her husband did have an affair. The procedural memory she would have constructed after the onset of her dementia would be that her husband was sometimes away from home, that it always seems like he is gone for a long time, and that he never tells her where he has gone, nor where he has been. She would construct this procedural memory based on her repeated experience of having her husband go shopping and not being able to remember what he told her about where he was going, due to her short-term memory loss, and not being able to estimate how much time has elapsed since he left. Her insecurity would build just from being alone. Under the same circumstances, if a person did not have dementia, an affair would be a reasonable thing to suspect. Figuring out a way to support her sense of security, rather than arguing time after time that you are not having an affair, will help this situation.

In another family, the lady with dementia could not remember that her husband was away three times a week for dialysis treatments. She also developed a delusion that her husband was having an affair. In this case, her husband made special arrangements to have a telephone available to him and found that his wife was much better when he called her to chat and reassure her two or three times during his treatments.

A delusion that their spouse is having an affair is unfortunately quite common amongst people with dementia. I included this in my standard teaching for spousal carers. Many spouses were greatly relieved to find out that this is a common occurrence, and to understand why it was happening. Dismay and embarrassment would otherwise have left them suffering in silence.

People who have dementia move through phases. For a few months they may be thinking about their work, later they may be worried about contacting their parents or their children or driving their car. It is helpful to write down the situations that you find yourself dealing with most often, and what your response is. It will help you organize your thoughts and you will be able to share the information with others who are involved in the care.

Short-term memory loss often leads to people misplacing things in the house and not being able to remember where they left them. If they are losing things in the house, they often have the delusion that the reason things are disappearing is because someone is stealing from them. "Someone is coming in here and stealing from me," becomes a procedural memory due to repetition of the experience of not being able to find something and thinking that it has been stolen. If you park your car in a certain spot, and come back to find it missing, you would immediately think it was stolen. You trust your memory and that is the best explanation for your car disappearing. People who have memory loss still have the life-long procedure or habit of trusting their memory. Thinking something has been stolen, because they can't remember where they put it, or that they were the person responsible for putting it somewhere, is a delusion. The delusion is based on a lifetime of experience of always being able to find things unless they had been stolen or moved by someone else.

Usually when we fear that something will be lost or taken, we hide it. When people with dementia hide things and then forget where they put them, it is frequently very difficult for anyone else to find them. Often carers would calm down the person with dementia who was agitated about the disappearance of a possession by saying they will help look for it and then doing so. One woman with dementia seemed to have an obsession for knowing where her purse was. She would very frequently lose her purse. Her family went out and bought four more identical purses in order to decrease the amount of time she spent in distress. She no longer carried important documents in her purse, but they were able to set up each purse with a change purse, keys and papers. When she lost her purse, they would go to where they kept the extras and give her one of those. When the one she had lost reappeared, they would tuck it away for the next time it was needed. This allowed both the family and their mother to cope with her symptom of severe short-term memory loss with minimal disruption to their day and minimal emotional upset caused by her delusion that she was the victim of a thief.

People with dementia are often unable to keep track of their finances, due to short-term memory loss and loss of abstract thinking, They may have the delusion that the reason they don't know how much money they have is because someone is hiding it from them. They may also be worried about their bills being paid. One daughter made a sign for the front of the refrigerator in her mother's house. On it she listed the bills that had come in, how much they were and that they had been paid. Her mother had been calling her many times a day to ask whether her taxes, hydro, water and other bills had been paid. When she did call, her daughter could ask her to go to the refrigerator to read the sign, and help her look for the item. Repetition of this process many times allowed her to develop the procedure of going to the fridge to look on her own. However, at the same time, this daughter also had to refrain from telling her mother how much money she had in the bank. If she knew she had any money, she immediately spent all of it on lottery tickets, without any thought to needing the money in the future to pay her bills.

Delusions are the logical consequence of a person with dementia not being able to remember everything about the context of their life. To give thoughtful dementia care in this situation means helping the person with dementia regain calmness and contentment, even though you will never be able to help them understand what is actually true.

2.L.ii. Illusions

Illusions occur when the person with dementia senses something, but their brain does not interpret it properly. One example, which was discussed previously, is that of the woman who saw a lady with a green dress in place of the small tree that was in front of her. It is often a challenge to discover these illusions and to work out what to do about them. The person with dementia may change their behaviour for a reason that no one can figure out easily.

Another illustration is that of a lady who suddenly refused to get into her bed. Her son was puzzled about why his mother began to sleep on the couch and would not sit on or lie down on the bed. She had never had such a problem previously. Her son began to think about the new comforter he had bought for his mother's bed, and realized that his mother's behaviour of not going to bed had started immediately after the new comforter went on the bed. His mother often chatted to herself about things that didn't always make sense to the son and he had developed the habit of ignoring the things his mother was saying, if there was no pressing need to understand. As he thought further, he realized that his mother had begun to talk about snakes around the same time he had bought the comforter. It took him quite a few days to figure out his mother's thought processes, but eventually he realized that his mother was experiencing an illusion that the stripes on the new comforter appeared to his mother to be snakes. You can certainly understand his mother's reluctance to get into bed. Why would anyone lie down with snakes on the bed? Turning over the comforter so the plain side was up was all that was needed, once the son had understood his mother's need. After that she had no objection to climbing into bed at night.

Another woman experienced the animation of objects with complex patterns. The figurines on her shelves and the flowered pillows on the couch became little animals such as dogs and cats that moved. She did not want to have these animals on her shelves and on her couch, so her son had to take them down and put them away out of her sight. Trying to talk her into the reality that these were not actually animals would have caused her great agitation. She had no control over experiencing them as animals in her reality, and helping her feel secure and unthreatened could only be accomplished by dealing with the situation within the context of her reality.

One fellow looked out the window into his back yard as it became dark. There were bushes being blown by the wind at the end of the yard. When he looked at them, however, he suffered an illusion that the swaying bushes were enemy soldiers with guns. He was a war veteran and had had similar experiences, so his fear was enormous. His daughter understood that he was having an illusion, and staying within his reality, wisely said, "Those are your hunting buddies." This reinterpretation of what he was experiencing made him feel safe, and he said, "Oh! I should go hunting with them again soon," as he left the room smiling.

A fellow who was a resident in a nursing home could very frequently be found trying to get out through a door that went onto a courtyard. The top half of the door had a large window. He spent hours trying the door and talking to himself, and banging on the door. Distracting him helped for a little while, but every time he walked by, he began again to try to get out. Everyone assumed that he wanted to leave the building. Trying to figure out how to help him, one person stood by him and listened to what he was saying. He was talking about his brother, who had died five years previously. Carefully observing the situation from the point of view of the person with dementia, the carers were able to put his conversation together with the fact that he was seeing his own image in the window. His need was not to leave through the door. He looked like his brother. He had the delusion that if he opened the door he would be with his brother, and he needed to see him. Covering the window with material that allowed light to come in but stopped the reflections led to an end to this behaviour, and likely decreased his stress considerably.

Illusions can happen with the senses of smell, taste, hearing, touch and proprioception, or the sense of body position and movement. One example of an illusion in the sense of proprioception was that of a woman who had a great deal of difficulty whenever she went for a long ride in a car. After a half-hour or so, she would start to call out "Why are we going up? We're going up, up, up!" Of course, the sensation of going straight up in the air under those circumstances would be quite frightening, and she understandably had a lot of fear. For a time, her husband found that she would calm down if he stopped at the side of the road for about twenty minutes. He would then be able to continue for about another half hour, until he again had to stop to let her calm down. Eventually, he had to stop taking her on long car trips.

The slowness of processing information can complicate the illusions that people have when riding in a car in busy traffic. If the cars and trucks are moving more quickly than the person's brain can process the information in their visual field, they may have the illusion that the vehicles are jumping from place to place. One family related how this had happened with their father and he eventually refused to get into any car at all. He would have established the procedural memory that all car rides are terrifying.

One person with early stage dementia eloquently described the illusions created by the slowness of processing. He said that when he put a coffee cup down on the table, he knew he had put it down, but he could still feel the weight of the cup in his hands, and could still see it in his hand. He also said that if he looked at a person and then looked at the other side of the room, the image of the person he had been looking at was dragged across the room as he turned his eyes. This was a person with a lot of insight who realized that the dementia caused by his Alzheimer's disease was causing him to experience these visual disturbances. If the same thing were to happen to someone who had no insight into their health situation, they would have had the illusion that one person was standing on the two sides of the room simultaneously, and it could be very confusing for them.

Another example was the lady previously mentioned who had the illusion that she was going up the stairs when she was actually going down. She had the insight to understand that she was experiencing an illusion. If someone without insight were to experience the same illusion, it would be very frightening. They may develop a procedural memory that stairs are frightening and then refuse to use them. This type of situation underlines the need to thoughtfully respect the wishes, and especially the refusals, of people with dementia. Even though their behaviour may seem incomprehensible to us, it is important to accept that within their context, they have a reason for acting the way they do.

2.L.iii. Hallucinations

Everyone's brain is able to create images and 'movies' with full colour, sound, touch sensations, smell and taste, and proprioception. We do this every time we dream. When explaining hallucinations to people I often asked them to recall the dreams they have when they're asleep, and then compared hallucinations to dreaming when wide awake. There must be a mechanism in the brain that prevents us from having dreams in a waking state, since that is the universal experience. It helps a carer to understand hallucinations if they think of that mechanism as being broken, and no longer preventing the person with dementia from having dreams, or hallucinations, while wide awake.

A few people described their family member as having hallucinations with the sense of smell. They would experience a powerful, and usually unpleasant odour. They found that the only way to help the person was to open the windows and air the room. Expectations do have an influence on the way hallucinations are experienced.

Can you recall having a dream and then, actually in the room with you, a telephone started ringing? Many people have had this experience. What frequently happens is that the ringing telephone is incorporated into the dream, and we dream that we are trying to answer the phone for a few seconds before we actually wake up. Just as dreams are susceptible to being influenced by outside suggestion, many family members have found that hallucinations are also susceptible to outside suggestion.

One daughter talked about standing on the sidewalk with her mother. Suddenly, her mother became alarmed, pointed a few feet away and said, "There's a tiger!" This would certainly cause a great deal of fear. Her daughter calmly replied, "That's a lovely little cat." With that suggestion, the hallucination changed and her mother said, "It is a cat. Now, why did I think it was a tiger?" The sidewalk was empty of any animal.

Hallucinations may be very frightening. These are the experiences that carers need to try to change by inserting suggestions. An elderly woman in a nursing home looked out the window at an empty parking lot. "Look at all those children lying on the grass!" she said. "What's the matter with them? Are they dead?" Her carer looked out the window, saw the empty parking lot and said, "They are having a lot of fun in that playground. They're on the swings and the slides." The lady cheered up, gave a big smile and said, "Oh! Isn't it nice to see those children having such a good time?" If she had been left alone to believe that she was seeing a field of dead children, this woman likely would have become very agitated.

One fellow was very angry at the strange man whom he frequently hallucinated in the apartment he shared with his wife. His wife noticed that through the course of his Alzheimer's disease the frequency of his hallucinations went in cycles. He would go for weeks not having any, and then they would start to occur once or twice a day. They would increase in frequency to a dozen or more every day, and then start to taper off again until he would reach a point where he had no hallucinations for a few weeks until the cycle started up again. Needless to say, she had many opportunities to try various approaches. She tried saying it was a friend. That didn't work because he demanded long explanations about who the stranger was and how long he'd known him. Of course, her first response had been "There isn't anybody here," but in her husband's reality, he certainly was there, so she got nowhere with that approach. One day in exasperation, she said, "He'll be gone in a minute." With that suggestion, her husband's hallucination ceased quite quickly each time, and he was satisfied. Things went well, until the day she came in tears, saying "Now he's seeing this man in bed with me! What can I do?" I said, "It's too bad you don't have one of those giant, man-sized teddy bears." "We do!" she replied. Her husband usually had this hallucination when he was coming back to bed after getting up to the bathroom in the middle of the night. After that, she called his hallucination, "the teddy bear" and agreed to move it so there was room for her husband in the bed, and, fortunately, he accepted this explanation. Very often, if someone came to visit, her husband would say, "Well it was so nice to see him, but who was that other fellow who sat in the other chair and didn't say anything the whole time?" She would say, "Oh, that's just his friend. It's strange that he was so quiet, isn't it?"

It is very thoughtful and kind to use this strategy of helping the person with dementia, who is hallucinating, to place their hallucination into a context that is acceptable and does not cause them to feel fear.

Carers do not need to reinterpret and make suggestions about those hallucinations that do not cause fear. Many people hallucinate visits and telephone conversations with relatives who have passed away many years ago. They have long happy hours with the relatives with whom they enjoy their hallucinated visits. Although it feels strange at first, many carers find they can easily get used to this situation. One lady was even able to laugh when she recalled that her husband offered her his imaginary phone, suggesting that she speak to his deceased mother. She was able to graciously decline the offer. It seems surreal to be living with this situation, but it's much, much better than argument and stress.

When people with dementia who have insight, discuss the things they hallucinate, the best approach is to openly call these 'hallucinations.' "Your brain is playing tricks on you and showing you things that aren't there; these are called hallucinations" was often an easily accepted explanation.

One woman came in with her daughters to find out about her own dementia. When I gently mentioned the possibility that she might experience hallucinations at some point during her illness, she was greatly relieved. "Thank goodness! I thought I was going crazy! I've been seeing angels and leprechauns!" She had never told her daughters about her experiences, but was very relieved to find that there was a medical explanation for what she had experienced so frequently.

Another fellow frequently saw animals in the house. Prior to being told about hallucinations, they agitated him. Afterwards, he would ask his wife if she could see them, and when she said she couldn't, he would calmly describe what the animals were doing. He had the insight to accept the fact that he was hallucinating and to know that his wife wouldn't lie to him.

Panic attacks were seen by one gentleman as the cause for his hallucinations. If he had some anxiety, he might hallucinate one or two strangers in the room staring at him. In a full panic attack, he would experience the room as being full of dozens of people staring at him in a disapproving manner. He knew that he was hallucinating these people even at the times when he was seeing them, but he could not prevent these hallucinations.

While visiting a couple in their home, I was told by the gentleman with dementia due to Alzheimer's disease, "I see people in our house all the time. My wife tells me that they are not real. She is a good woman, so I think that she's probably telling me the truth." Distraction and thinking about something else often results in the hallucinations disappearing. Interestingly, this fellow had evolved his own procedure for getting rid of the hallucinations. He no doubt noticed that if he went to the bathroom, the hallucinated people in the house were gone when he came out, as his thoughts would have been focussed on what he was doing in the bathroom. This became a procedural memory for him and then he turned it into a deliberate procedure for himself. "I don't mind if there are one or two of these people around, but it gets so crowded if there are dozens and dozens of them and I get tired of it. So I go into the bathroom. Sometimes I don't even do anything when I'm in there, but when I come out, they're gone!" He was triumphant at having conquered this annoyance for himself.

Invariably, family carers who are being asked "Where do all these people come from?" when there is no one else in the house, are dealing with delusions stemming from frequent glimpses in mirrors on the walls, or people who are being hallucinated. Taking down or covering the mirrors to see if it helps is a way to identify if it is a delusion. Trying to identify what type of situation is occurring just before the hallucination starts may help to decrease the likelihood of the person with dementia having the hallucinations. However, for the most part they seem to be spontaneous and not triggered by any external event. Calm reinterpretation and distraction each time were the best approaches developed by carers.

In one instance a fellow, would frequently say to his wife, 'Alison,' "Where's the other Alison?" He seemed to be conscious of the fact that he frequently saw her and another lady exactly like her. In another particularly complex instance a fellow was seeing multiple copies of his wife, who we shall call 'Marg' for the purposes of this story. Not only did he see them, but also each of these hallucinations was talking to him and moving around independently of the others. He had very limited insight into his situation. If he accompanied his wife to the grocery store, he would express his worries to his wife. He would say to her "What about Marg? We left her at home. She needed to get groceries too!" It is possible that the slowness of processing visual information contributed to this experience and that as she moved, her image would stay where it had been in his mind. It seemed more likely to happen if she was moving quickly, preparing meals or trying to be fast when she was doing her housework. Staying calm and quiet with very little activity seemed to help him come out of this distressing situation.

A child crying was the hallucination that one woman heard over and over again. Her carers remembered her talking about a time in her childhood during World War Two in Europe when she was very sad and cried a lot. They wondered if what she was hallucinating was the memory of herself crying. Comforting her was the only way to help, not telling her that she was imagining these sounds. Naturally, telling her that it wasn't real was the way they first tried to deal with the situation. This is a normal thing to do and carers learn by trial and error that contradicting the belief of the person with dementia usually leads to more upset and agitation.

Some family carers found that the severity and frequency of unhappy or stressful hallucinations was decreased if their physician prescribed an antidepressant or an atypical antipsychotic for the person with dementia. Combined with thoughtful care, this may help. However, such medications may worsen the person's ability to keep their balance or to stay awake during the day, so their use needs to be very carefully evaluated. People with Lewy Body disease, who have many hallucinations, are unusually susceptible to severe reactions to such medications. There is further information about these reactions available from the Lewy Body Dementia Association (www.lbda.org). Each case is unique and the balance between help and harm is difficult to find. Making every attempt to live with the situation without added medication avoids the side effects and reactions that medications may cause. However, at times the situation is so severe, that side effects must be risked in order to bring relief from an intolerable situation. Living in these circumstances can be emotionally painful for the person with dementia, and doing whatever can be done to ease their burden of suffering without making their condition worse is often the aim of health practitioners and family members. As the disease causing the person's dementia progresses, there may no longer be a need for medication. After a few months, a trial of decreasing or stopping the medication will be useful to see if it is still necessary.

3. Losing the Functions of Everyday Life

3.A. The Progression of Dementia

After the initial stage of a progressive degenerative neurological disease causing dementia, the progression of the disease causes damage in other areas of the brain until the damage is global, involving the whole brain. The abilities that each individual retains at any one time, depends upon the unique progression of the disease in their brain.

The constellation of inabilities that a person has is determined by the location in the brain where the disease started and the course of its advance. Different diseases affect different abilities at the beginning. Alzheimer's disease typically begins with short-term memory loss. Changes in judgement usually appear first with Frontotemporal dementia. Parkinson's disease starts in the motor area of the brain, causing tremors and difficulty with movement, and may or may not progress to a dementia in other areas of the brain. The first symptoms of Lewy body disease commonly include hallucinations. Some people have more than one of these diseases that cause dementia, further complicating the understanding of their symptoms.

The initial symptom of Vascular Dementia will depend on what area of the brain has been affected by the stroke or the many small strokes the person has suffered. The location of a stroke depends on where the blood clot or blood vessel rupture happened in the brain, that is, where it caused brain cells to die because they were deprived of oxygen as a result. Our brains are organized geographically. Everyone has the same general area assigned to control of all the functions we do whether it's walking, writing, talking, singing, doing arithmetic or any of the other host of things that we do.

Not every stroke progresses to dementia. Changing lifestyle habits by avoiding or controlling diabetes, stopping smoking, exercising regularly, losing excess weight, and keeping blood pressure and blood lipids (fats) within normal ranges will help prevent the progression of strokes into Vascular Dementia. The brain is also 'plastic.' Sometimes when people have had a stroke, they are able to relearn the function they have lost because a different area of the brain takes over that function. This requires lots of trying and failing and practice to allow the brain to create new brain cells and new pathways between brain cells in order to establish a new ability. Norman Doidge wrote a fascinating and easy-to-read book called "The Brain That Changes Itself" which describes brain plasticity.

Progressive neurological degenerative diseases cause continuously increasing damage in the brain until death. Regaining of functions with brain plasticity has not been found to occur with the dementias caused by progressive neurological diseases such as Alzheimer's disease, Lewy Body disease, Frontotemporal dementia or Parkinsons's disease with dementia. However, following a healthy lifestyle of a good diet, exercise, lower stress, and sufficient engagement in activity is thought to slow the progression of dementia in some people. Although there are dozens of diseases that cause dementia, together these four diseases plus Vascular Dementia are the most common and account for almost all of the individuals who have dementia.

It is very difficult for a doctor to diagnose exactly which disease is causing the dementia because the symptoms overlap, and it may be difficult to know in what order they appeared. It is too dangerous to do a biopsy of the brain as it can cause so much damage. Most of the time, diagnosis is made on symptoms only. Scientists are working to find blood tests and tests of the fluid around the spinal cord that may help to support a diagnosis of the specific neurological disease that is causing a person's brain to degenerate. Most brain scans are not detailed enough to help with a diagnosis early in the disease. Blood tests, which are done during diagnosis, are to look for other medical problems besides a degenerative brain disease. Other medical problems could cause the symptoms of delirium that appear to be dementia, or may worsen the symptoms of the dementia.

3.B. Changes in Physical Abilities

Until this point, it is mainly the changes in thinking processes that have been discussed: the immediate, short-term, long-term, procedural and emotional memory processes, the speed of processing, selection of which part of the environment to which to pay attention, and the changes in interpretation of sensory information. However, the brain also controls and coordinates all of the movement of muscles in the body. As the person's condition deteriorates with the advance of dementia, their physical abilities also decrease.

Dementia due to Alzheimer's disease and other degenerative diseases affects muscle strength and coordination. It is typical for the change in physical abilities to begin with fine movement such as a deterioration in the accuracy of small movements of the hand. This may be seen in the first few years as shaky handwriting. People may seem to be clumsy as they have difficulty grasping and holding onto objects. Other tasks that require precision with hand movements may also be difficult. Lack of depth perception may increase the effect of clumsiness. For example, if the person is trying to pick up a glass of water, they may knock the glass over as they reach for it. Small movements that have always been automatic, such as picking something up, are lost as the procedures for those activities are forgotten.

In addition to fine motor movement, the dementia also affects the movement of large muscles. The most notable change is a lack of strength to walk for a longer period and to walk quickly. In particular, it is difficult for people with dementia to take long strides, and as their disease progresses their steps become shorter and they need more frequent rest periods. The ability to balance is also affected. As this happens, the person develops a slow, shuffling walking gait and starts to become prone to falls. They may walk with their feet far apart to stabilize their balance.

In the late stages of dementia, the ability to walk is lost. Similarly, the person loses the ability to direct their arm movements, and their strength may be greatly diminished. In the late stage the large muscles may have a strong contraction, particularly if they are emotionally startled or stressed. This is often experienced when the carer is dressing the person with dementia. You may need to pull their arm or leg out from their body in order to put on a piece of clothing, only to have it pull back from you. You may form the impression that they are being uncooperative. However, they do not have that intent and are unable to control this contraction of their muscles. As they rest, the contraction will release on its own in a matter of minutes.

3.C. Loss of Complex Functions

Although the type of functions lost initially depends upon which disease is causing the dementia, there are general patterns that everyone with dementia has in common. The ability to plan and organize tasks becomes severely compromised early in dementia because of changes in memory or judgement. The person with dementia begins to lose the ability to start off, or initiate, the movements designed to accomplish a particular task. As any person continues with a task, they need to perform a pattern of movements skilfully and in the correct order. This is also disrupted by dementia.

People with dementia gradually stop being able to look after the daily tasks of their household activities such as shopping, preparing food, repair, cleaning, and gardening. The ability to do simple, one-step tasks lasts longer than those that require many steps and careful planning. As their dementia progresses, their need for assistance also progresses. There are many illustrations of these changes.

The more complex the function is, the more it depends on many different areas of the brain working together, at the same time. Complex functions such as using the telephone, driving or arranging transportation, shopping, food preparation, housekeeping, managing medications, doing hobbies, being active in community groups, working, and managing finances, are lost early in the dementia process because they rely on so many areas of the brain to function. If one area is not functioning, the person is no longer able to perform the function at all.

These complex functions are sometimes called 'executive' functions because they require a number of different memories, different skills and the ability to understand the sequence of each of the steps of a procedure and their relation to the other steps. Say, for example, there are fifty areas of the brain involved in doing a task. If only forty-nine of those areas are able to work successfully, the person may not be able to do that task or may do it badly. Performing duties around the house becomes impossible for the person with dementia, even though they appear to be physically capable of carrying out those duties. Take the example of boiling an egg. One must know what an egg is, that boiling it requires putting water in a pot, heating it to a boil, and leaving the egg in for the correct amount of time. If any one of those steps cannot be performed adequately, the person with dementia cannot boil the egg.

The person with dementia may be able to do things for a period of time if the steps are broken down for them. For example, if you say "please put these plates on the table" and then later when they have finished with the plates, you say, "please put these forks on the table," you have done the planning and organizing that they can no longer do. If you had said, "please set the table," they would have had to remember all the steps and the different items required. For a period of time, the person with dementia may be able to copy the steps and method of doing a task if they work side by side with another person doing the same thing; but eventually, this too, becomes impossible. By the way, because of changes in the understanding of where the things are, and where they should be in space or on a surface, the table is likely to be set in a disorderly and disorganized manner. Their willingness to help and what they have accomplished should be praised. Thoughtful dementia care means that the person with dementia will not be humiliated by being criticized or teased for doing a messy job.

The picture is complicated because the person with the dementia has good days and bad days, and, for a while, they may perform the required function on some days but cannot on other days. There may also be times when they spontaneously do a task correctly even though they are incapable of doing it when asked. It may seem as though they are refusing to do the task, but it is much more likely that at that particular instant, they are not able to understand what is wanted or are not able to do it.

As mentioned in the section on the changes in long-term memory, the use of a telephone is an example of a household function that we may use many times a day. You need your long-term memory to remember what object is called a telephone and how to use it. You need your short-term memory to remember the person you are calling, the number you are dialing and the reason for your call. You need the brain to properly start and to control the large muscles of your hand and arm to get the telephone and to hold it. You need the brain to coordinate the small muscles of your fingers to press on the number buttons. Your long-term memory holds the knowledge of how to find a telephone book and how to look up their number. Your brain needs to be able to receive the visual information from the telephone directory, interpret it properly, and focus clearly on the tiny numbers. If you are calling a business, you may be given a series of many choices to press numbers that correspond to the service for which you are looking (even people with an intact short-term memory find this process challenging). You need language skills to speak and to understand what is said to you. Your brain needs to be able to process the information you are receiving quickly and respond quickly by initiating and controlling the muscles of your face and the muscles you use to control your breathing and voice box to make the sounds needed to produce words. All of that is needed to make a 'simple' phone call.

Many people with early stage dementia would say to their callers, "Slow down please. I have dementia." They found that this was very helpful in letting them have a successful phone call.

One fellow had a full sized piece of lined paper. On every one of the thirty or so lines his mother had written out the same phone number. She had crossed off each individual digit, probably trying to remember which of the seven numbers she had already dialed and which came next. Some lines had all the individual digits of the phone number crossed out, some only a few. One can picture a determined, but frustrated, lady, very bravely trying to overcome the effects of her disease in order to make a simple phone call.

Another family set up a phone with a large red button on the side that would call an emergency number when pushed. The fellow with dementia was able to remember this procedure. However, he had developed another procedural memory: whenever someone asked him to practise using the red emergency button, he could never find it. The solution to this problem was to turn the telephone a quarter turn so the side of the phone was facing him. After that was done, he said, "THERE it is!" He had lost the capacity to remember where the button was when it was out of sight.

When trying to use the telephone, most people with dementia start to have difficulty with looking up numbers first. They then become unable to dial and may only answer the phone, but not make calls themselves. They often forget to pass on messages. Later they may not be able to use a telephone at all. Telephones that are equipped with small pictures of family members, and will speed-dial the corresponding phone number with the press of one button, may lengthen the person's ability to use the telephone for a year or more (these phones are available at http://alzstore.com, and may be at other places as well).

Cell phones are difficult for people with early dementia to use because they forget to charge them. Changes in visual processing and fine muscle movement may make it difficult for them to dial the small number pad. Their use is so recent that if a person has difficulty with the last ten years, or so, of their long-term memory, they may have lost the knowledge that it is possible to have a phone in your pocket or purse with no wires attached to it. This lack of knowledge may cause them to be startled and become agitated when it rings.

Cutting the grass became the only outside chore for a man who could no longer garden. One day, his wife did not hear the lawnmower start up, so after a few minutes she went to investigate. Since the last time he had cut the grass a week earlier, her husband had forgotten how to turn on the electric lawnmower. Once she turned it on, he was able to cut the lawn.

Another fellow had the job of putting the garbage out every week. He came to his wife one day because he couldn't find the garbage cans. She didn't want him to feel badly, so she said, "I just moved the garbage cans to the garage," even though that is where they had always been kept.

Another man was able to put the garbage cans and recycling boxes out at the street, but was not able to judge when to bring them back. He would frequently take the cans and recycling boxes back to the garage, even though the garbage hadn't been picked up and they had not yet been emptied.

A lady whose husband had dementia related that the last year he planted the annual flowers in their garden, they didn't do very well. At the time, she was aware that he was watching what she was doing, and copying her movements as she planted another flowerbed beside his. The next spring, she discovered that, in the sequence of steps to plant the seedlings, he had neglected to remove them from the plastic seedling holders, so they were root-bound and failed to thrive.

The preparation of food requires the abilities to plan multiple steps at the same time, and to hold them in the memory for a long period of time. The items to be used in the meal must be purchased at the store, usually by driving there. People with short-term memory loss will have difficulty with the shopping as they may not remember to put all the items on their list, and may come home without some of the items even if they are on the list. They may also have difficulty handling money or remembering all the steps required to use a credit or a debit card. Their judgement about what to buy may be greatly affected and they may spend far too much money.

The steps that are required to make a meal are housed in the long-term memory and also in the procedural memory. If you imagine someone setting out to make a sandwich, they would have to remember to assemble the bread, spreads, filling and greens on the counter and then use a knife with skill and precision to complete the preparation.

Concentration was an issue for one woman with Alzheimer's disease. Her family thought she wasn't able to prepare food and she argued that she could. As it turned out, when they were with her, they would stand in the kitchen and chat as she tried to cook and she could no longer concentrate on both chatting and cooking and she wasn't able to complete the meal. After the family members understood that interrupting her with conversation while she cooked was an unfair test, she was still able to make lunch while they waited in the other room.

Remembering the steps was the issue for another lady whose dementia was more advanced. Her husband was trying hard to encourage her to keep active. He would lay out the ingredients of a sandwich on the counter and watch with sadness and frustration. He timed her at over an hour, picking up and putting down the knife and moving the ingredients around on the counter, without making any progress at getting the sandwich made. He was having a great deal of difficulty accepting that his wife could no longer do the chores that she had been doing for over fifty years.

A daughter whose mother's dementia was progressing very rapidly expressed her disbelief at the skills her mother had lost. Twelve months earlier, she had been able to prepare an elaborate meal for over a dozen family members. This year, during the same celebration, she had sat in a chair while everyone else did the preparation; she had become unable to make something as simple as toast and tea. It is more typical for this amount of deterioration to take place over a few years.

In addition to the other stresses of having a family member with dementia, the carer who remains healthy often has to learn to take over the role that has been abandoned. Spouses (mainly husbands) who have never cooked need to learn how to make meals. Others (mainly wives) need to learn how to maintain a car or how to manage finances. One lady had to ask her minister for help. He showed her how to write a cheque, as she had never written one before her husband was no longer capable of doing it. Other spouses have been unaware of such things as the location of the air conditioner in the house, the fact that the furnace filter needed to be changed, or that oil changes were needed for the car. It depends on how the work of their household was organized before the onset of the dementia. If their roles overlapped, it was easier to fill the other person's shoes. One fellow was irritated because his wife, although she could no longer do the laundry, hovered about when he was doing it, telling him what to do and criticizing him if she thought he wasn't doing it properly. It is difficult for people with dementia to give up doing the things that they have always done. I asked him, "If you were the person with the dementia and your wife was out trying to trim the hedge, do you think you'd be telling her how to do it?" He grinned, as he understood that he certainly would have been trying to get her to meet his own standards of perfection in the tasks that were normally his to do.

It is challenging for a person with dementia to do laundry. When this happens to each individual is unique. Understanding that the clothes are dirty, knowing how many clothes to put in the washing machine, how much soap to add and how to set the dials are functions of the long-term memory and the procedural memory, and mistakes may be made that end up ruining the clothes or not getting them washed at all. With short-term memory loss, people who are still capable of doing laundry may forget that they have put a wash on, and discover it many days later, wet and smelly, still in the machine. For a time, some people are able to cue themselves to remember that they have a wash going, by placing a laundry basket in the hall. Eventually, however, they will be unable to remind themselves why the basket is there in the hallway.

Housekeeping and home maintenance also require multiple skills and memory processes to be used at the same time. People forget how to perform the tasks, and what they have already finished. Their judgement about what should be done is also lacking. One lady said that she vacuumed the entire house every week. She was not lying; she truly believed that what she said was true. Her husband had a different story. She could still get out the vacuum cleaner and get it started, but she would spend an hour or more vacuuming the same corner of the living room, and then put the vacuum cleaner away, satisfied that she had done the entire house.

One family had complete confidence in their father to make house repairs, only to come home and find that he had drilled many, many holes in the walls. He had definite intentions of putting up a shelf, but suddenly had lost the capacity to do more than drill the holes.

Although they are losing many functions, people with dementia may continue to try to do the tasks they used to do because they want to feel useful. It is important to make it easy for them to find something to do that satisfies their need to accomplish goals. One lady saw that her husband, who used to be able to fix anything in the house, performed only one task. He would wipe down the kitchen sink and counter for hours with a cloth. She provided suitable cloths for him in the kitchen, on top of the counter where he could easily find them, so that he could continue to be proud of the fact that he was contributing and staying busy. He was not able to judge that his activity was actually not helping much at all, but he had peace of mind, nevertheless. Such activity may not usefully contribute to the management of the household, but it is very useful in providing contentment for the person with dementia.

Knowing which abilities remain and which inabilities need to be compensated for is important for carers. It is difficult to step into the personal space of someone with dementia and take over a function when they are no longer able to do it. They may do it one day and not the next. They may be offended because they feel they are still capable of taking care of things themselves. Using good humour, showing respect and caring, trying and failing and trying again, the carer eventually helps the person with dementia get used to the fact that they need help. Further deterioration means that the carer needs to start this process all over again.

If the person with dementia has been responsible for maintaining relations with the rest of the family, arranging get-togethers and hosting gatherings, someone else in the family will need to take over this role. If connecting, either by phone or through visits, has always been initiated by the person who now has dementia, other members of the family need to be sure that connections still happen with the same frequency. Family gatherings may have to be moved to someone else's house if the activities of the preparations are overwhelming to the person with dementia. Both during the preparations and during the gathering, one person at a time may need to be designated to keep the person with dementia occupied, to work alongside them as they do whatever they can to help prepare, and to keep them calm and relaxed. If the person with dementia finds these preparations overwhelming, this may mean going for a walk or a drive to get them away from the activity. If no one is assigned to the person with dementia, their anxiety may build without anyone noticing because the family members are concentrating on their own activities and their own conversations.

3.D. Driving

Driving a car is a very difficult thing for a person with dementia to give up. When they stop driving they become dependent on others to take them places. If they live in a rural area where there is no public transportation, driving is a necessity to purchase food and other household goods. If they live alone or their spouse does not drive, losing their driver's licence causes a major crisis. In many communities, driving is essential in order to visit stores and go to entertainment events and restaurants, or to visit with friends and families. However, in a city, there are more options. Friends and family may live nearby, groceries and drug prescriptions can be delivered. In a city, it can be less expensive over a year to take taxis a few times a week, than to make car payments along with purchasing insurance, repairs, gas and licences. Spontaneous car travel, which is very much enjoyed by many drivers, is no longer possible in either the city or the rural areas, when journeys must be scheduled with others. Even though it may be available, independent use of public transportation is not suitable for people with dementia because of the risk of geographic disorientation when using it. One family received a call from the city transit authority to tell them that their mother would ride on the bus around and around the circuit. Each time she took the bus, the driver would eventually have to help her get off at her stop by asking to see her identification and looking at her address and figuring out which stop was hers. Of course, they were worried that once she got off the bus, even if it was at her bus stop, that at some point she would get lost trying to find her way to her home. When people with dementia are sent by taxi to a day program, the staff insists that they are accompanied into the room where the program is being held, as many have gotten lost if they are left on the sidewalk outside the building and expected to find their own way to the program. Consequently many day programs have had to develop their own transportation service to bring their clients to their program.

While there are transit services in some communities for disabled people at a reduced rate, those services often exclude people with cognitive disabilities. The funding is so restricted that there would not be enough service for those with physical disabilities if the criteria for qualification for the service were broadened. People with dementia would also need room for two because they would have to bring a companion to help avoid becoming lost after they've reached their destination. Volunteer drivers are usually available only for medical appointments, but not shopping. These situations will differ from community to community. What is true in every community is that if we need people to stop driving because of the onset of dementia, there need to be reasonable alternatives for them to access. As it stands now, there are frequent stories about people who refuse to get a medical assessment concerning their dementia, because they do not want the doctor or the Ministry of Transport to have reason to take away their driver's licence. The testing that they may be required to take in order to keep their licence after diagnosis costs hundreds of dollars, and this is another reason people who suspect they have dementia resist bringing it to the attention of their physician.

There are many changes that occur during the progression of dementia which have a detrimental effect on the person's driving skills. Slow processing of sensory information by the brain leads to people reacting more slowly when the situation in traffic changes; they have increased reaction time. Geographic disorientation leads to people with dementia hesitating when they are behind the wheel as they try to figure out which way to go. Lack of depth perception makes it difficult to tell how far away the curbs and the other cars are.

Many people with dementia also have spatial disorientation. They can confuse left with right, backward with forward and have difficulty understanding how objects are placed relative to each other. This can cause great difficulties when driving. A gentleman, while he was driving on a four-lane road, thought he was in the right lane when he was in the left and vice versa. This led to him making right hand turns from the left lane. One woman parked between two cars that were in adjacent parking spaces. They were far apart, but there was no marked parking space between them for her car. She managed to do it without damaging the cars, but she and her son could not open the doors, and he had to coach her to back out to choose another spot. Both of these families realized after these incidences that their loved one with dementia was no longer safe to drive a car.

Misinterpretation of numbers means that posted signs of speed may be ignored, as will numbers on a speedometer. One fellow consistently said he was driving at forty kilometres per hour (kmh) when the speedometer read seventy or eighty kmh. He was quite certain that he was driving within the speed limit, when he was not.

If a person with dementia has lost the long-term memories for certain sounds, they may not pay attention to the sound of cars honking, or the sound of another car's engine as it approaches them from behind. Failing to recognize traffic signs and signals could lead to these being ignored. There are many stories of people with dementia becoming involved in traffic accidents as a result of such inabilities.

Decreased peripheral vision means it is harder to see when cars are approaching from behind to pass, as well as seeing pedestrians and bicycle riders who are nearby. One fellow said he had no difficulty turning left, but whenever he had to turn right, he ran his car up on the curb. This was directly related to his decreased peripheral vision. When he turned left, he was able to use mainly his visual field that was directly forward, but when he turned right, his lack of peripheral vision caused him to misinterpret his position relative to the curb.

Short-term memory deficits lead to an inability to multitask. It is necessary when driving to always know what is in front of you, what is behind you, how far away from your destination or your next turn you are, where there are lights and crosswalks and bicycle lanes. Driving is a multitasking function and requires an intact short-term memory.

Sometimes during testing, a physician will find that the person's spatial skills are such that they need to cease driving immediately. Other times, the family may want to curtail the person from driving, because when they sit in the passenger seat while the person with dementia is doing the driving, they find their driving unsafe. Sometimes people who suspect they have dementia or who are told that they do, voluntarily give up driving immediately as they realize that their condition endangers their own life as well as that of others should they get behind the wheel.

If a person with early stage dementia is continuing to drive, it is helpful for family members to arrange to be a passenger about once a month, in order to see if they continue to feel comfortable being driven by that person with dementia. When they reach the point that they are no longer comfortable, then the process to help them give up driving should be started. In order to be a fair assessment of how they are when they are driving alone, the passenger should not chat or distract the driver in any way, in order to see how they are driving when their full attention is on the road.

It is worthwhile remembering that people with dementia may forget that they are not permitted to drive. Keeping the keys out of sight, rather than hanging on a hook by the door, will make it less likely that they will mistakenly go for a drive.

This is an issue that can make powerful emotional memories in a person with dementia. I met quite a few people with dementia who could tell the story about how they lost their driver's licence years after it had happened. Favoured children who suddenly insisted that their parent never drive again found that their parent would no longer speak to them and this would continue for months and years. Taking time to meet with other family members and devising a way to help the person with dementia cease driving with minimal emotional trauma can avoid many pitfalls. There are many resources to assist in this process. One of those that is quite helpful is the website of "The Hartford" insurance company which has information about driving with dementia and a booklet and DVD that can be ordered to assist in the process of driving cessation by the person with dementia.

This situation will test your patience. Try to be thoughtful of the crisis this represents for the person with dementia. Never vary from being gentle, kind, understanding, and reassuring, no matter what angry words are aimed at you. This crisis will pass, and you are both less likely to have any lasting anger from going through it, if you consciously avoid unpleasant arguments in the first place. The anger that may come from the person with dementia is part of their own grieving for the fact that they are going through this dreadful illness and losing their abilities, and their freedoms, and so much of what has given their life meaning.

4. Losing the Ability for Self-Care

Eventually people with dementia will lose the ability to care for their own cleanliness and grooming. When this will happen varies among individuals during the course of their disease progression. Since these skills were among the first learned in the individual's lifetime, they will be among the last lost in most people with dementia. People do differ in the development of their symptoms, depending on what areas of the brain are affected at any one time, but 'first in, last remaining' is the general rule. The reference to the research conducted by Barry Reisberg, which established this pattern, can be found in the section entitled "Suggested Readings, References and Resources."

Grooming, bathing, and personal care are disrupted when the person forgets how and when to do things. They may forget what the steps of washing are because of the loss of the memory of the procedure. They may forget that they need to wash. They may be unable to remember how much time has elapsed since they last washed or changed their clothes due to their short-term memory loss. They may lose the long-term memory that regular washing is necessary and expected. They may also believe that they are clean and take offence should anyone suggest otherwise. Dealing with such situations in a manner that is kind and jovial, rather than confrontational, is important.

Helping a person with their personal care means invading their personal space. Giving personal care is especially intrusive, and trust must be established each and every time that the person with dementia is approached. This is made more difficult if they do not realize that they are not properly groomed or dressed and are not maintaining their former standards of cleanliness. They may reject any help given as unneeded and annoying, or even as an attempt to physically attack them. Great care must be taken, using a kind and thoughtful manner, to slowly get them used to, and accepting of, the new procedure of receiving help in the care of their person. Confrontation is painful and disruptive for both the person with dementia and the carers.

Faced with such situations, many people have hoped that there is some way to 'get through to the person with dementia;' to make them understand what is true and what is not true. The tragedy is, of course, that this does not exist. There is only slow, quiet reassurance, establishing a new procedure in small steps, with warmth and kindness that will make it possible for the person with dementia to use their procedural learning ability to feel safe. Carers are encouraged to 'take baby steps,' to help them understand how slowly they need to make changes.

4.A. Dressing

Getting dressed starts with the realization that one needs to get dressed or change clothing. To choose what to wear, it is necessary to know what time of day it is, what is appropriate to wear at that particular time, and what is suitable for the weather outside. To accomplish the next step in getting dressed, a person must be able to decide which specific items will fit their needs. Following that, a person must be able to manipulate the buttons or zippers, understand how the clothing goes on their various body parts and then be able to make all the appropriate physical movements while keeping their balance. Loss of any one of these memories or abilities will interfere with the ability of the person with dementia to get dressed. During this process, the person with dementia may be distracted, and, because of their short-term memory loss, forget that they are in the middle of getting their clothes on and do something else. Before they start, they will also have to face the similar challenges of first getting undressed.

Looking at a closet of clothes is rather similar to looking at a restaurant menu in terms of the decision-making process that is required. What is appropriate for the weather or the occasion? Which top matches which bottom? What else do you need besides the top and the bottom? If a person with dementia does not remember what is in their drawers, a sign on the front of the drawer may be helpful, if they agree to have the sign. It is necessary to be specific, using labels such as "bras" or "boxers" rather than the general abstract category of "underwear" which they may no longer understand includes items such as briefs or panties, bras, shorts or boxers, socks or undershirts. It is best to use whatever term they have always used for that item of clothing. If you ask, "can that sign be read easily?" it is less insulting than "can you read that sign?" A picture of the item could be placed on the front of the drawer for a person who is no longer able to read.

For most people with dementia who are having difficulty, the first step in helping them with dressing may be to choose what they will wear that day. Somewhat later, the carer may realize that the person with dementia is uncertain of the order in which to put on their clothes, so the carer needs to change their strategy by laying out the clothes in the order in which they are to be put on. They choose whether the order will be from the head of the bed towards the foot, or the opposite, and once they have established that procedure, it should not change. Knowing what order the clothes go on means the person with dementia needs to be able to know where to start and what piece is next until they are completely dressed.

As their dementia progresses, the person with dementia may no longer be able to look at a piece of clothing and understand whether it goes on the lower half of their body or the upper half, or, whether it goes next to their skin or it is part of the outer layer of clothing. If you know whether they have always dressed the lower half of their body first, for example, it will help to use the same order when you are laying out the clothes. If the procedure is changed after it has been established, the person with dementia may still put the clothes on according to the old system, and then they will not be properly dressed. Later on, the person with dementia will need help in being handed the clothes in the correct order, and eventually they will need help putting on the clothing and doing up the buttons, zippers, belts and other fasteners.

The geographic disorientation that happens in dementia, which starts with an inability to orient themselves in their community, in their neighbourhood, and in their own home, eventually extends to disorientation to their own body. Think of a small child learning what their hands are, what their arms and feet and legs are. Later the children learn how to orient their limbs in order to put them into clothing. So, if you think of a toddler just learning to dress themselves, and then push the thought back to before that stage of development, you will arrive at an understanding of the adult with dementia who loses one skill after another in putting on their clothes.

Forgetting the geographic layout of their body, general loss of long-term and procedural memories, and loss of planned, skilled, and coordinated muscle movement all contribute to a developing inability to dress. People with dementia demonstrate the loss of this skill by often putting their feet into sweater sleeves, or putting things on backwards. Looking at the different parts of the clothing, they can no longer make sense of where their limbs are to go, or whether the garment is back to front or upside down or what part of their body it is designed to cover or whether it is an inside or outside layer.

How to make the appropriate movements to cooperate with help in getting dressed is also lost. For example, one fellow became unable to cooperate with his wife as she dressed him because he forgot that he needed to raise his foot off the ground in order to get it into the trouser leg. Instead, he pressed his foot into the ground. He remembered that there was something he needed to do with his foot, but pressed down instead of pulling up. His wife at first thought he was being uncooperative on purpose, but then realized that she had to change her tactics and have him sit to put clothing on his lower body. As with a very young child, the appropriate movements required in dressing are not known. At some point, a carer will have to pick up their loved one's hand or foot and place it in the clothing.

People with dementia often get grumpy about their need to accept help with personal care. This is completely understandable since they are grieving the loss of their ability to be independent and may feel that it is unjust to be treated like a small child. It is therefore important to respect their adulthood and not use the type of nicknames or baby talk that we sometimes do with small children while helping them with dressing or any other personal care tasks. One carer discovered that if she gently said "Good job!" to her husband with dementia, over and over again during the day, it was the most helpful approach to his ongoing frustration.

Each individual is different. Some accept help easily, even wondering out loud what took the carer so long to help, and some don't. One lady found that if she asked her husband if he needed help with his shirt or told him he needed help, he found this very upsetting. She found that the best way to approach him, with his need for help and his unwillingness to accept it, was to wait for fifteen to thirty minutes, letting him try over and over to put his own shirt on. When she felt it was the right time, she approached him without speaking and gently helped him with his shirt. His pride was badly hurt by having to accept help to dress. If he had also had to request help or say yes to her offer to help, it was as though that doubled the hurt to his pride. So it was important for her not to ask him if he wanted help. It may also be suitable for the carer to approach and start to give help while talking about something entirely different. What suits each person with dementia needs to be established by trial and error.

The patience and acceptance needed on the part of the carer is enormous. For whatever reason, people with dementia do not usually say "thank you" for the help they receive. Perhaps it is because they are grieving deeply for what they have lost. They need so much help, that they would be saying "thank you" every few minutes or more often. Part of helping them maintain their self-esteem is to stop expecting this rule of politeness, in order to have the constant help they need seem like a normal part of everyday life. Because they seldom get thanked, I have told many carers that they need to stand in front of the mirror occasionally, and say to themselves, "You're doing a great job!" Giving care to a person with dementia is very important and reflects the essence of human virtue and kindness. Knowing and reminding yourself of that helps your own self-esteem. Be proud of yourself.

Often the circumstances in which the carer needs to give help are extremely challenging. One lady's continuous occupation was to rearrange her clothing into drawers or containers all over the house. She did this all day long with great energy. It kept her fit and active and her husband did not interfere with her need to do this constant rearranging. However, in addition to all the other help he needed to give her to dress, he also had to try to find the clothes that she would be wearing, never knowing where he would find them from one day to the next. He was gentle with her; however, he did need to express his frustration, and anger at the situation he was in, to other people who understood what he was experiencing.

One family was extremely upset when their mother, who had been diagnosed with Alzheimer's disease many years before, began removing all her clothes repeatedly. This woman had always been very proud of the way she dressed, and would have been mortified to be naked in public, if she had still had her former judgement skills. A solution was found when the staff at the nursing home, where she resided, used a one-piece bathing suit as her undergarment. The bathing suit had a strap added across her upper back that she could not undo. Consequently, when she removed her clothes, she remained decently covered by the bathing suit.

Some people with dementia develop a very strong procedural memory in which they will only wear one outfit. This makes it difficult to wash their clothes. The family of one lady who insisted on wearing the same green track suit everyday, finally found that their best tactic was to go out and buy five identical green track suits so she could be clean at the same time that she was comfortable in the way she was dressed.

Track suits are very easy to put on and take off. Once carers start to have difficulty with helping the person get dressed, they often abandon the fancier clothes and stop struggling with nylons or other complicated undergarments. Many families I knew helped their loved one with dementia change clothes only once in twenty-four hours, in the morning or the evening, depending upon when the procedure was easiest. They completely abandoned the idea of wearing pyjamas to bed as it meant another difficult dressing session, and the people with dementia in those families stayed in their clothes to sleep.

A lady whose family had started to dress her in track pants found that she was continually looking at her legs and running her hands down her thighs to her knees, saying "This is terrible, terrible!" over and over again. She was very distressed. When they learned about the change in memory processes, they remembered that she had always worn dresses and skirts and had often said that she thought that it was wrong for women to dress in trousers like men do. When they put an apron on her that tied around her waist and ended at her knees, she no longer showed this distress. Looking into the person's past for a clue about their distress can be very helpful.

In many instances, it is the emotional pain being suffered by the person with dementia that can be eased by thoughtfully making a small change in their care. Figuring out what change to make often requires careful thought and problem solving with others to generate ideas about how the person with dementia is experiencing the situation and what is causing them distress. It is sometimes helpful to think of ways to help the carers if they are experiencing emotional pain and distress. In the example of the lady who was clothed in a bathing suit, her family's need was met without severe restrictions or consequences to their mother. This was a problem for them, not her, and in this instance, altering her care on their behalf was appropriate. If their mother had become agitated and angry whenever she was approached to put on the bathing suit, that should have been taken as a clear refusal of that element of her care, and they would have needed to seek a different solution.

Thoughtful Dementia Care:
Understanding the Dementia Experience

4.B. Bathing

Over the years, I met couples who were comfortable being in the bathroom together, others who had never once been in the bathroom at the same time in over fifty years of marriage, and many whose comfort level was somewhere in between those two practices. If you have never been comfortable being together in the bathroom, you will have to either learn how to overcome your discomfort or make arrangements for someone else to give the intimate care that will be required. If you are an adult child, or another relative or friend, becoming comfortable in the area of giving personal care is even more difficult. Eventually, the person with dementia will need the same amount of assistance that is required by a very young child.

A very slow (over weeks) invasion of the personal space of the individual with dementia is a comfortable method to use. The first step might be to leave the door open yourself when you go in to wash your hands or face. You could also chat to them from the hallway about other things, to get them used to you being present in their private moments. Then if you follow them in to just get something before they shut the door, and gradually take longer and longer to leave, eventually you can just stay, and neither one of you will think it is remarkable.

One fellow related how he would always ask his wife to wash before dinner. One day she didn't return to the kitchen. When he went looking for her, he found her at the bathroom door. She knew she had to go into the bathroom to wash, but she couldn't remember what to do to wash. At this point, it would have been important for him to allow his wife to avoid embarrassment or humiliation. Avoiding humiliation in this example might be done by picking up the soap, smelling it, handing it to her while you turn on the tap, and then washing your hands together. It means that you are not confronting the person with dementia directly and verbally about the fact that they have forgotten how to wash. Staying calm is difficult when presented with a shocking new development like this. If you can't stay calm, skip the washing and eat dinner anyway, until you have time to recover and plan your next move. Dementia does not always allow you to follow the rules.

Understanding the difficulties that the person is having often means reviewing the changes in memory processes and then carefully examining the situation and the environment of the room in which it is happening. One fellow, who needed to help his wife bathe as she was no longer able to do so herself, was puzzled because she had been calm and cooperative with his assistance for months. Then she began to become agitated after he helped her step out of the bathtub, and wanted to get covered up immediately. Initially, it seemed to him that he had not altered anything about the bathing procedure and he couldn't comprehend her sudden change in behaviour. However, her dementia had progressed and she had developed an inability to understand mirrors. As soon as she saw her own reflection in the mirror, she thought there was another person in the bathroom, and she was embarrassed and anxious. Once he covered the mirror, she did not become upset when he was helping dry off after her bath. The cause of the distress for a person with dementia is not always readily apparent to the rest of us, who can take intact thought and reasoning for granted.

Many people with dementia are reluctant to bathe, especially when it comes to having water pour over their head and face. If this happens, it is important to accept those feelings and to be careful about not letting water wash over their face, and talk to them about how careful you both need to be as you are doing it. It may help if you hold a wash cloth over their forehead, or have them hold it if they are able to cooperate, as this will help prevent water from flowing over their face when their hair is being rinsed.

Many people have difficulty getting the person into the tub or the shower in the first place. Avoiding talking about the bath directly may allow them to be more accepting. Being direct means the carer is saying, "It's time for your bath." Being indirect may be something like, "Your bath water is run. Do you want to use the pink towels or the green towels?" or, "As soon as you are finished your bath, we can go out for an ice cream cone." or "Here is some aftershave lotion that you can put on after your bath." Making the bath acceptable may include saying, "We both need to have a shower before we go to the store. Do you want to have yours first or second?"

Slowly getting them used to your presence in the bathroom while they bathe, will also let you observe whether they are actually thoroughly washing themselves. "Do you want me to wash your back?" may be a good entry to actually giving 'hands on' help with the bath. For a long while, they may retain the ability to do the motions required for actually rubbing the washcloth on their skin, but need help with the step of getting the cloth wet and putting soap on it. Although they may lack the ability to plan and to wash themselves with purpose, it is quite common for people with dementia to imitate their carer by copying their movements and washing the carer's arm or face.

One fellow, whose mother had a great deal of difficulty getting his father with dementia to bathe, took him to his gym and they both showered there. His Dad was quite comfortable with this arrangement and could probably relate to post football or soccer games and practices when the whole team would shower before changing.

There are many ways to stay clean besides standard tub baths or showers. The aim is to keep their skin from breaking down because of contact with body fluids, or with food that has lain on the skin. Many people use a shower chair and a showerhead with a long hose attachment to allow more control over where the water goes and to help the person who cannot stand in a shower because their balance and stamina are decreased. Family members will sometimes wash the area between the person's legs, also the area most prone to skin breakdown, when they are just getting up from the toilet or when they are standing and leaning against the bathroom counter. Even bathing in bed can work. Putting plastic underneath the sheet that they will lie on, to protect the mattress, and, keeping every part of their body covered and warm except the area being bathed, may be pleasant and much easier if they are reluctant to bathe in the shower.

Because of short-term memory loss, the person may forget what is happening when the two of you are part way through a task, such as a bath. Gentle reminders or a 'play by play' monologue helps some people: "Now I'm washing your foot, and I'll just get in between the toes. Now I'll dry that off before I wash the other foot....." People have found it effective to keep chatting like this throughout the task, as the continued connection and reassurance of a soothing tone helps the person with dementia stay calm in a situation they would otherwise find threatening.

If the areas that can develop skin breakdown are cared for well, the person may not need a full bath any more than once a week. Many people use dry shampoos that stay in the hair in between hair washings, or trips to the beauty parlour or barber shop. There are also troughs that are specially designed for washing a person's hair in bed, in which the water drains off the side into a bucket. Great efforts of creativity are needed in the trial and error process to find a bathing method that is acceptable to both the carer and the person with dementia.

Having a distraction can be helpful. Talking about the dog, or even having it in the bathroom during the bath to make the distraction more successful may work. Music, talking about the person's life in grade school, anything at all, can be the topic of conversation. The procedure needs to be pleasant, with laughter and relaxation. This will support the development of a procedural memory of a bath that is fun and not accompanied by fear and panic.

Keeping the bathroom very warm is important. We expect to get a little chilly because we are wet, but a person with dementia may not connect the cold they feel with the fact they are wet, and especially with the need to put up with being cold in order to be clean and waiting for a few minutes until they can be warm again. If they are cold, they want it to change so they can be warm and nothing else matters because they are not thinking about two things at once.

As with all functions with which you must help the person with dementia, it is important to find out what has changed for them, which step in bathing they are having difficulty with and what they can still do for themselves. If you take over the steps that they can still perform, it decreases their self-esteem, their feeling of usefulness and their pride in being able to do things for themselves. Also, if their muscles are not kept active doing these personal care tasks, the loss of whatever hand and limb movements they have left will be hastened. However, it does take longer when they do it themselves, without a doubt.

Gradually, this personal care is no longer what you do to get ready for an activity, but it takes so much time that it becomes the activity for the morning. If you find that the time moves too slowly for you, perhaps listening to music or a talking book with earphones would help you.

If you have any way of getting someone else in to help with the morning care so you can pursue your own activities, this will give you great relief. As with other changes, slower is better. Ideally the new carer should be consistent, not a different person each time. There is too much about each individual with dementia that must be learned in order to keep them feeling secure. Having a consistent carer who comes into the home, may also allow the person with dementia to build a procedural memory of them. If you have the new carer observe you, allowing the person with dementia to get used to their presence, they will gradually accept their care. Many people introduce professional carers as friends of the family. The person with dementia cannot comprehend and empathize with the strain that giving care puts on their carer and their need for relief. The presence of their main carer is their security and they are likely to panic when that person leaves. A gradual transition will allow them to get used to a new procedure while maintaining their sense of personal safety.

One fellow with dementia was very upset when a paid carer began to come to their house. He became more agitated with each visit, and he was getting close to pushing her back out the door. His wife then repeatedly put a small bag of his favourite candy in the mailbox. When the paid carer came, she brought the candy in, saying, "Look what I brought for you!" Later she took pictures of his dog and helped him put them up on the fridge. His procedural memory changed so he understood her visit as something enjoyable. Over many weeks, she was able to slowly gain his trust to let her help with his personal care.

Many long-term care facilities are using a care method called Gentle Persuasive Approaches, which can be very useful in accomplishing care procedures such as bathing. There is a web address for this program in the section entitled "Suggested Reading, References and Resources."

4.C. Toileting

The ability to toilet oneself is also affected by the changes in dementia. There are many thinking processes whose deterioration may lead to a lack of success in toileting and the development of incontinence or 'having accidents.' Full incontinence does happen in the late stages of dementia. However, there are many ways the carer can help the person with dementia make up for some of the abilities they have lost, that will help the person stay accident free for longer.

If a person can no longer find the bathroom due to geographic disorientation the carer can figure out the best way to help them. I have mentioned the lady who put a picture of a hockey player on the bathroom door. Her husband was able to understand his need to find the toilet and verbalize a request for help. Other people with dementia will wander about the house and not ask for help. Whatever method they used to use to find the bathroom is no longer working for them and they need help finding a new procedure that will work.

Using contrasting colours may help. An example of this would be to paint the door a colour that no other door in the house is painted. To establish the procedure they can be led to the door for many days until you see they have established the new procedure in their mind and go there themselves. Leaving the bathroom light on at night may help draw them there when they get up during darkness. A night light outside the bedroom door may help them return to bed.

Some people put signs up in their house. It is important to work out an agreement with the person with dementia beforehand and ensure that they can read the sign. Others will take a picture of the toilet, and put that on the bathroom door. It is also important to make sure that no one who is visiting will remark on the sign and make fun of the need for it, as this can embarrass and upset the person with dementia so much that they may insist the sign is taken down.

At a different time, perhaps before the issue of geographic disorientation inside the house arises, it would be helpful to distinguish the doors that lead outside and to establish the procedure in the mind of the person with dementia by talking about it every time you both leave the house. This may help prevent them from accidentally leaving the house when they are looking for the bathroom. An example of this would be to paint or put a picture of the same flower, or tree, on each door that goes to the outside. Make sure it is a picture that you can live with, as you cannot change it without depriving the person with dementia of the procedure they have learned. Each time you go outside, you draw attention to the picture, saying something like, "I love the picture of the maple tree that is on each door going outside." If your loved one with dementia has sufficient insight, they may be able to work with you to establish this memory.

Other people may start to develop incontinence because they can no longer connect the feeling of a full bladder, or pressure from their bowels, to the need to find a toilet. In this instance, developing a procedure in which you take them to the toilet automatically every two hours or so may be effective. That practise will make sure their bladder does not get too full. There is a sphincter, which ordinarily prevents the urine from leaving the bladder until we let it go, but that sphincter will automatically release to empty the bladder of urine when the capacity of a person's bladder is exceeded. Older men often develop an inability to feel any pressure in their bladder until it is almost too late to make it to the bathroom. If they also have dementia, it makes the same situation that much more complicated.

Most people have a usual time every day when their bowels move. Keeping track of this and making sure they are led to the bathroom at that time can help ensure bowel continence. Eating a meal or having a hot or cold drink often stimulates bowel movements. Knowing these characteristics for the person for whom you are caring will help you find the best way to assist them. Raising their feet on a low stool while they are on the toilet also makes it easier for them to move their bowels.

A deterioration in the skill with which the person can move their hands and manipulate their clothing may mean that they have an accident while they are still trying to undo buttons or zippers in order to use the toilet. They may need your help with the fasteners on their clothing. This is one of the reasons people start to wear track pants; there are no buttons or zippers that need to be undone. If the person with dementia is wearing an incontinence product, it is easier for them to manipulate pull-ups, rather than those with tape fasteners.

Changes in the muscle coordination of the legs and in the long-term memory may mean that sitting is now difficult. If they are weak, a high toilet seat may help. They may need to use a grab bar beside the toilet to help themselves sit down and get up again, and this will save wear and tear on the carer's back and shoulders. If they do not remember how to sit down, they may need to be coached each time to turn their back to the toilet, back up until they can feel the toilet at the back of their legs and then bend their knees. If their sense of depth perception is such that they cannot figure out their position relative to the toilet, having an outline of feet on the floor and coaching them each time to place their feet there before they sit may be helpful.

Being unable to remember to use toilet paper, flush the toilet, wash hands (knowing the steps of turning on the taps, getting the soap, scrubbing, and drying the hands) as well as being incapable of performing the needed muscular skills, in the correct order can also affect a person's ability to be continent. Knowing what skill has deteriorated and what they can still accomplish requires close observation and problem solving on the part of the carer.

Contrasting colours are helpful to compensate for a deterioration in the ability to distinguish objects in the environment and a change in depth perception. Painting the wall behind the white toilet a darker colour will help the person who has difficulty seeing a white toilet on a light coloured wall. Following the same idea, using a coloured tub mat will help someone see the bottom of the tub, or a few drops of blue food colour will help make the water in a white bathtub visible. Commercial toilet bowl cleaners that stain the water blue will help the person aim for the water, if they are standing, or to find the seat if they are trying to sit down. However, even taking these steps, one lady reported that she still had to clean the floor around the toilet several times a day, because her husband could no longer aim properly. She thought about getting him used to sit down to urinate, but decided against that route. She reasoned that since he had lost so much already, she was not going to deprive him of the manly dignity of standing to use the toilet.

Short-term memory loss may mean that the person forgets that they were trying to find the bathroom or that they are in the middle of using it and they may leave before they are done. Thinking up a way to keep them there until they finish requires some creativity. One such creative carer sat on the edge of the bathtub and sang duets with his wife until she was finished on the toilet. The person with dementia may also be distracted by the presence of mirrors, which will further detract from their ability to stay concentrating on their task.

Eventually the person with dementia loses control of the sphincters, the round muscle groupings that open and close to allow the bladder or bowel to empty. Both the person with dementia and the carer will be helped by the use of incontinence products. Fortunately, these are now made in many styles to suit adults. This usually happens in the late stage; however, on occasion it is an early symptom of dementia. If a person, who has usually toileted themselves, becomes acutely ill, with pneumonia, for example, they may become incontinent for a time and then recover. However, usually incontinence is permanent once it develops. Getting financial assistance for the purchase of incontinence products may be possible. Their cost may be eligible as a medical expense on income tax, they may be available from a food bank, or various charities or other family members may be willing to assist.

Many family carers have related how they have searched around town, finding the restaurants that have family bathrooms, and choosing those because they are able to accompany the person with dementia into the washroom. Otherwise a man or woman might be unable to follow the person with dementia who is the opposite gender into a public washroom. A few people were pleased to relate how they had received help from a store clerk who closed the needed washroom for everyone else temporarily, in order for the carer to avoid the embarrassment of being in the wrong one. Occasionally, kind strangers helped out by going into the public washroom to make sure the person with dementia was alright. Very often carers kept a change of clothing in the car, in the event that it was needed.

It is very important for the carer to maintain an attitude of acceptance and a pleasant manner when dealing with this sensitive element of personal care. If the carer complains or makes comments or facial expressions that are negative, the person with dementia may respond to the disapproval by becoming uncomfortable and anxious in any situation in which they require assistance with toileting.

4.D. Mobility

As mentioned in the discussion of changes in physical abilities, mobility becomes decreased by dementia when the areas of the brain that control muscle movement and coordination are affected by the dementia. The skills that require the movements of the small muscles of the hands are ordinarily affected first. Think of how you use these muscles in everyday life: to brush your hair and your teeth; to use toilet paper; to pick up eating utensils such as knives, forks, spoons, or chopsticks, or to pick up the food directly with your fingers; to write and to type; to fold laundry; to make the bed and hang up your clothes; to use a shovel, throw and catch a ball or to pat a pet or drive a car or a bicycle. When the use of these muscles is no longer available to the person with dementia, it means that there are many things that they can no longer do. Some of those functions will be taken over by other people, and other functions will simply be lost, because the carer cannot possibly do everything that another person used to do and all of their own functions as well. Getting the person with dementia used to accepting help with such activities requires the approach of using baby steps in making small changes, trial and error to see what is successful, redesigning the methods of care as their abilities change, and maintaining a warm and friendly attitude that promotes the feelings of partnership and mutual cooperation.

Changes in walking include decreased stamina. The person with dementia gradually becomes less able to walk long distances, and less able to walk quickly. They have a tendency to shuffle: taking small steps without raising their feet off the ground. As well as walking with their feet far apart, many people with dementia try to improve their balance by holding onto furniture or touching the walls. Complicating the issue of balance loss is the fact that the person with dementia may not remember that they are prone to falling and will try to get up to walk on their own, despite being asked to stay sitting until the carer returns.

If a person with dementia does start to have frequent falls, they should still remain freely up and about. People who are using their legs regularly keep their muscles developed and are less likely to harm themselves if they fall. Keeping a person with dementia mobile for as long as possible should be a goal of care. Immobility for just a few days will cause rapid deconditioning in a person with dementia and they may need regular help until they regain their ability to walk. Restraints should never be used. Imagine that you are tied in a chair or a bed. There is no one around to help you, no matter how much you call out. You are terrified. This is inhumane, and decreases the health of the person. People with dementia who were subjected to restraint in the past were more prone to pneumonia and skin breakdown, including deep ulcers. Many, in struggling to get out of restraints, have twisted themselves about so they end up dying from strangulation by the restraints. For further reading on this issue, there is a reference for an article by V.T. Cotter in the section entitled "Suggested Reading, References and Resources" at the end of the book.

If a person is falling, it is important to look for a reason besides the progression of their dementia and a decrease in stamina or strength. Changes in the environment can protect or endanger the person with dementia. One woman received a call from the long-term care home in which her husband was a resident to say that he had started falling a few times a day. This surprised her because his habit was to continually walk with a shuffling step most of the day, only occasionally stopping to sit on a couch in the lounge. When she went to the home, she walked behind him, observing that his walking did not seem any different. However, when he got to the lounge, he went straight to an empty spot on the floor and sat down on the floor. This was the place where the couch he had always sat on had been. The staff had decided to rearrange the furniture in the lounge, not realizing that he had such a strong procedural memory and a lack of problem solving skills and judgement that he would sit down on the bare floor, in the same place, regardless of the fact that there was no longer any couch to sit on. Once the couch was put back where it had been, he had no more 'falls.'

People with dementia can be taught to use a walker, and then sometime later also taught the proper way to walk inside it using the spaced retrieval method mentioned earlier. Establishing this habit when it is needed is important. I have known many carers who have developed repetitive strain injuries in their shoulders and backs because they were spending hours every day supporting the person with dementia to walk and to get up and sit down. The person with dementia may be able to help themselves with grab bars in the bathroom. They may need the carer to coach them each time to grab onto the bar. A bed assist rail can be used by the person with dementia to help themselves get out of bed. Asking a physiotherapist or occupational therapist for the best way to support the person physically without hurting them or yourself may prevent injury.

Many carers used a plastic garbage bag on the car seat to make it easier to adjust the position of the person with dementia on the passenger seat. They may be unable to shift or slide themselves toward the centre of the seat, or unable to lift their legs into the car and pivot into a forward-facing position. Care must be taken that they don't slip off the seat when getting out.

When people with dementia become completely immobile, it may take two people, or one person with a special hydraulic lifting apparatus, to get them up from the bed to the chair. Normally, we change our position frequently during the day, without thinking about the fact that we are preventing the damage to skin and underlying tissue that continued pressure can cause. At this point, people with dementia will no longer make the small shifts in position that are needed to prevent the area of their skin that is under most pressure from being deprived of circulation. Small shifts every thirty to sixty minutes or so will prevent deep tissue damage and ulceration that can result from unrelieved pressure. These pressure ulcers can also develop from sitting in the same position in a chair without regularly shifting. Any area of the body in which the bones are close to the skin surface develops pressure ulcers more easily. Special mattresses or mattress covers with alternating pressure mechanisms can be purchased. Most people with dementia are being cared for in a long-term care home by this stage, and the staff will have regular procedures to prevent such injuries.

4.E. Eating

Disruptions in eating due to dementia are quite variable. People forget whether or not they have eaten and neglect to eat, or they may eat too often. They become unable to make judgements about whether they are hungry or thirsty. Their ability to taste food changes, as they lose their sense of smell. As dementia progresses to the late stage, many people experience difficulty swallowing. Safety concerns arise if the person with dementia lacks the judgement about what is food and what is not. In this situation, household poisons such as bleach, laundry detergent, turpentine and others may need to be in a locked cupboard.

I have known a few people with high anxiety, who continually paced the floor, and getting them to sit to eat was almost impossible. Carers in these circumstances often found that leaving a nutritious bite-sized snack on a plate where the person with dementia would notice it as they walked by, meant that they would grab it and eat it as they walked. Often they got more nourishment into them this way, than they had before when they spent most of their energy trying to get the person with dementia to sit down on a chair at the table and to stay there long enough to eat something.

Consider an instance of a person who has lost the ability to feed themselves well, has lost the knowledge that a certain feeling in their stomach means they are hungry and need to eat, and, has lost the ability to understand most words. They are fed a couple of bites, and, seemingly have lost interest in eating. Their short-term memory does not allow them to remember that they are in the middle of a meal. They may not recognize food as food, or connect it with the task of feeding themselves. Someone asks them if they are full. They may hear what sounds like nonsense words – sjopm flrtem wdber – for example. However, wanting to be polite, they may answer a raised inflection in the person's voice with a socially acceptable "yes." This results in their food being taken away before they have had enough to eat. People with dementia reach a point where others have to take on the task of assessing whether they have had enough, as they are no longer able to judge their own nutritional intake for its adequacy. They may feed themselves once they get help starting, or they may need to be fed by someone else. They may not recognize feelings of thirst, and may go without drinking for long periods, or work outside on hot days without taking in adequate fluids, risking dehydration.

Some people with dementia may overeat, as they fail to recognize the physical feelings of fullness, do not remember that they have just eaten, or are no longer able to exercise their judgement to give themselves adequate nutrition. In some instances, keeping food out of sight, or not having inappropriate food in the house is the only way to cope with a person going through this type of phase. This can cause real conflicts for a carer. In one

Thoughtful Dementia Care:
Understanding the Dementia Experience

instance a lady had to stop having her delicious cookies and squares available for her grandchildren, who adored them, in order to help her husband who had diabetes and Alzheimer's disease, but was no longer able to exercise appropriate judgement in stopping himself from eating as much as he wanted to eat. This caused grief to this carer, as she was no longer able to dote on her grandchildren in a way she and they loved.

When a person with dementia also has diabetes, it is very challenging to help them control their intake and their blood sugar. One woman's family became very frustrated because they had placed the diabetic teaching guide right on the fridge, and she was not using it. They would talk to her and explain to her what she should eat. She would study the guide carefully, and then open the fridge and eat the first thing she saw, whether it was carrots or a cake, seemingly ignoring all the guidelines. Looking at the fridge, it was obvious what her difficulty was. The instructions used abstract categories: for lunch she was to have a carbohydrate, a vegetable and a certain amount of protein. Even though her dementia was quite early, the instructions needed to be written in concrete terms, which specifically named the food, such as one carrot, one apple, one slice of ham and one slice of bread, rather than the general food categories. Better still would have been to prepare her lunch, and leave it on a plate at the front of the shelf so it would be the first thing she would take out of the fridge.

Many people described calling from work, and waiting while their family member heated their lunch in the microwave, sat down and started to eat it. The families had realized that this was necessary because so many days had gone by when they would come home at the end of the day, to find that the person with dementia had successfully heated the food in the microwave, but had forgotten to take it out and eat it. Similarly, one family member I knew called across three time zones every morning to stay on the telephone while her mother got a glass of water, took the pills that were left on the counter by another family member who was at work, and reported them to be swallowed. If you call only to ask if they have eaten, or what they ate that day, people with dementia will use their procedural memory to report the kinds of foods they can remember eating in the past. They want to reassure their family that they are fine, but the judgement and the short-term memory loss prevent them from being accurate.

Talking your way into managing the fridge of someone with dementia can be seen as an invasion of their privacy and a judgement that they are no longer capable of managing themselves, both of which are true, but highly insulting in their view. Taking small steps to get them used to having someone else go into their fridge to check for food that is past its expiry date, or to make sure that meals, which have been provided, have been eaten, is necessary to gain their trust. Family members realize that prevention of food poisoning takes precedence over hurt feelings, but even so, they will often remove food that has gone bad when the person with dementia is unaware. Many also have discovered that it is not enough to put it in the garbage, as people with impaired judgement have often been known to take it out of the garbage and put it back into the fridge, wondering out loud why anyone would want to waste perfectly good food. Instead, things that are thrown out need to be completely removed from the house for disposal.

Alcohol intake is a situation with which many families have difficulty. Drinking alcohol may further compromise diminished mental functions. Some doctors give permission for their patients with dementia to have one drink a day. However, the loss of the short-term memory may mean that they have forgotten they have already had their single drink, and they may repeat the process. One lady found that whenever her husband walked by and looked at the highball glasses in the china cabinet in the dining room, it triggered him into wanting an alcoholic drink. She packed all the glasses away in boxes and put them in her basement. In her china cabinet she placed her china figurines instead. Once he no longer saw the glasses, her husband almost completely stopped asking her for an alcoholic drink.

Eventually in the late stages, people have a wasting away, when they become very thin before they pass away. Using food supplements or favourite foods to get them to take in sufficient calories becomes the priority. People who are having difficulty swallowing are sometimes given tube feeding. This is rarely used in Canada for those who have late stage dementia, as it is widely viewed as prolonging their suffering and their dying process.

5. Staying Active

To help the person with dementia stay active, you can adapt your own activity when you are with them. A person with dementia needs to have their activities simplified. This may mean that you keep track of the complexities of a situation, while assisting them to do one step at a time. Everything can then be made to look clear and straightforward to the person with dementia, but you may be working very hard to accomplish that.

The person with dementia might be able to experience less anxiety during outings if you can keep them oriented, in the moment, to what is happening. This means that you slow down your own thought processes and think out loud, to keep yourself from making those mental leaps that the person with dementia cannot make. For example, if you are going to the grocery store, instead of silently parking the car, getting out and heading for the entrance, you could do a play by play: "Here we are at the store. The best door to go in is that green door ahead of us. The carts are here (as you point) on our right. Do you want to push the cart?" It is as though you are functioning as their stream of consciousness. If you find that the person with dementia is becoming anxious or agitated when you are out together, this may help.

This chatting, which keeps them oriented in the moment, eliminates the need for the person with dementia to remember where they are in the moment and to put it into the context of where they are going next. You are managing the complexity of navigating, while they are still benefiting from the stimulation and exercise of a shopping trip. The chatting will also give them another way to know where you are. Otherwise, they may get distracted, look at something else, and then experience a building anxiety when they realize they can no longer see you.

Signs are helpful to keep the person with dementia independent and active for a longer period. If a person with dementia is living in a multistorey retirement home, they may be going down to lunch. In order to get to the dining room, they need to get on the elevator and go to the second floor. It is helpful if there is also a sign in the elevator that says 'Dining Room' beside the '2.' Without that, people with dementia may get off on the wrong floor, wander around trying to find the door, get back on the elevator when they find it again, and go through that process a few times until they get to where they are going.

The more information that's available, the easier it is for the person with dementia to find their way around. On the same theme, if all the apartment number signs on the doors were coloured shapes, this would help the person with dementia navigate more easily. For example, this could mean giving the apartment number signs on floor three a red circle background and all the apartment number signs on floor four a green square background, and also putting the same colour coding on the numbered elevator buttons and the apartment keys. Further, if each person had a different decoration on their door, such as a picture of an iris, or a dog, it would help them identify their own apartment. It will take a few weeks for a person with early dementia to learn what the picture is on their door, so the individual's door picture should not be changed as long as they live there. Therefore, you could have a person with dementia who can no longer make sense of numbers, which is usually one of the early losses, pushing the button with the red circle on the elevator and looking for the dog's picture and successfully finding their apartment. They can build a procedural memory with that information, but not with numbers that they can no longer understand and interpret.

A person with dementia slowly loses the ability to plan an activity, carry it out step by step and evaluate how they are doing and when they are finished. They gradually need more and more help with organizing any activity and with 'hands on' help in completing it. Eventually, their participation may be merely observing. However, even observing is valuable, if they are engaging with the activity and with the person who is doing it.

People with dementia are very individual in what they find to be fulfilling activities. One person, who has been assisted to plant seeds, will hover over the seedlings all day, day after day, and find this fulfilling. Some enjoy going for a drive every day. Others may read the same page in the same book over and over again. Some enjoy walks; others would rather sit on their porch. Some people enjoy being with family and friends; others are only comfortable with just one other person present. Often the same activities are repeated many times. There is emotional security to be found in having the same familiar procedure repeated in an expected way, when so much else is unpredictable and unknown.

People with dementia find comfort in having something that is predictable and known. If someone has worked with a particular set of tools for much of their life, they may find comfort in just handling those tools, day after day, without doing anything 'useful' with them. The carer may need to revise their concept of usefulness. Useful may no longer mean that those tools are used to make anything, however they are very useful in bringing peace and contentment to the person with dementia who finds comfort in holding them.

One family was in a dilemma about whether to continue to permit their mother to access the barn on the family farm. All the children in this large family acknowledged that their mother still retained her long-term memories, ingrained since childhood, of how to safely navigate around the various hazards in the barn. They called this being "barn smart." She no longer had the capacity to do any chores, but wandered around in the barn

Thoughtful Dementia Care:
Understanding the Dementia Experience

many times a day and was very content there. Half of them felt she should be allowed to continue to go to the barn, the other half were worried about an unusual event or a deterioration in her condition that would cause her to have an accident at some time in the future. Their father wanted his children to make the decision. I asked them to try to connect with what her values would have been. If she had somehow been able to see into her future and had been asked to make the decision with all her faculties intact, would she have decided to play it safe and be prevented from entering the barn or removed from the farm, or would she have decided to live at risk, by continuing to wander through the barn she loved to visit? The decision of the children was immediate and unanimous. They knew that if their mother had been able to make the decision herself, she would have chosen to continue to wander in the barn with all its familiarity and associations of the memories of her past.

The way a person with dementia spends their time is very different than it was before they developed a disease causing dementia. They no longer need to finish what they are doing, whereas previously they may have been driven to complete the task and accomplish something. They may enjoy a card game, but the rules now need to be flexible. It is the process of playing and engaging with someone else that is important, not the goal to win or complete the game.

Flexibility on the part of the carer is very helpful. One woman described a card game that she and her husband continued to play in the early stage of his dementia. They had always decided at the beginning of the game whether they would play 'Jacks high' or 'Queens high.' However, after he developed dementia, he could not keep track of which was the high card for that game, so they decided that 'Queens' would always be the 'high' cards and never varied it after that.

Some carers will try new things they think the person with dementia might enjoy and that they would enjoy too. One daughter enrolled herself and her mother in a beginning pottery class. They had a lot of fun working with clay and being creative together. Some people with dementia who have never painted have found great pleasure in taking up a brush and creating something on canvas. It is important to shift your attention away from the things the person with dementia can't do, and look at things they can do and the verbal and non-verbal communications that you can share.

At any point in time during the period the person is living with dementia, it is important to know what activities they enjoy, what is too hard for them and makes them feel inadequate, and what they find too easy and would be humiliated if you suggested it. Many people feel that activities that children would do are too undignified for the person with dementia, because they are adult. However, they have the capacity to choose. If they pick up a doll and enjoy carrying it around, or if they pick up crayons and enjoy colouring, why should they not engage in this activity that is now fulfilling to them? They may not have made that choice before they had dementia, but find it engrossing and comforting in the present time. If you think there is an activity that they might enjoy, leaving the materials for it out, or doing it yourself to see if they are interested may be a gentle way to encourage them without being direct. Taking a walk around a craft store, hobby shop or toy section to see "what's new," would give you an opportunity to see what attracts them.

Many spousal and family carers are so busy with looking after their household and the physical and emotional care that the person with dementia requires, that they cannot imagine having time for recreational activities. However, every time they participate with the person with dementia in helping them through their daily routine, they are creating activities and assisting the person with dementia to remain active.

Some people with dementia need to be very active, and may restlessly pace. One family found that their mother with Alzheimer's disease responded well to having a rocking chair. She rocked with great energy, but it helped her fulfill her need to keep moving. I have often thought that putting automatic rockers on the bed of a person with dementia, who is no longer mobile, would provide movement that may be comforting.

Noticing what the person with dementia enjoys doing, and leaving out the things they need, will help them spend time in their comforting routines. An example of this is the previously mentioned lady who left out old tea towels on her kitchen counter so her husband with dementia could rub and shine everything in the kitchen for long periods, which he frequently did. The books by Jitka Zgola and Oliver James, mentioned in the "Suggested Reading, References and Resources" section, provide excellent further reading in this area.

6. Stages

Many family members are anxious to know what 'stage' in the disease the person with dementia is currently experiencing. The desire to know this is very understandable. They want to know how much time their family member will be living and what the next few years of their own lives will bring in order to plan for the future.

There are two elements to the answer. The first is to get a feel for the rate of deterioration. If there are changes from month to month which are noticeable to the carer who is living with the person with dementia, then the rate of progression is faster. When changes are noticed only every six to twelve months, then the rate of progression is slow. The changes that happen very slowly may only be noticed by people who see the person every few months. These deteriorations happen so slowly that the carer who is there every day often accommodates to them without consciously realizing it.

The average time for people to live after diagnosis of Alzheimer's disease is eight years. Lewy Body disease usually progresses a little more rapidly than Alzheimer's disease. However, there is a great deal of variability. People with Alzheimer's disease may live as short a time as two years after diagnosis, or as long as twenty years or more. If there are other diseases, such as heart disease, kidney disease, cancer, diabetes or other major conditions present, it can shorten the length of time that the person will survive. Temporary illnesses such as influenza may hasten the deterioration of the person with dementia. They will usually regain some lost abilities when they recover from a temporary illness, but they will not regain everything they lost. Having a temporary illness or a procedure such as a surgical operation may also change the overall rate of deterioration.

The second element to the answer about what stage the person is in depends upon what abilities they still have. There are many professional measurement tools, which measure such things as remaining language or memory, but the information they produce is not always helpful to family members. For example, knowing that a person can no longer draw a clock is very useful in helping a physician make a diagnosis, but it does not help family members who are trying to compensate for the inability of the person with dementia to tell time. However, I usually gave families a copy of the Clinical Dementia Rating Scale, which is freely available online. This scale gives a reliable estimate of the degree of dementia that is present, providing it is not used during an acute illness. Families often filled out assessment forms, for their physician, of 'activities of daily living,' which are used to rank how independent a person with dementia is in performing the skills that we all need to take care of ourselves from day to day. Family members could also use such assessments to evaluate whether their loved one with dementia had help in every area where it was needed, and to see what kind of help they may need to offer in the future.

The staging that many families found helpful was stated in terms of what the person with dementia would require in terms of assistance. In the first, or early stage of this simple three-stage classification system, the person is living at home, able to do simple tasks and able to communicate partially. The carer may be still involved in some activities outside the home that have nothing to do with giving care. In the middle stage, all the activities of the carer are centred on the care of the person with dementia in the home, and they may require help from other members of the family and outside agencies. In the final stage, the person with dementia is no longer able to be cared for at home because their needs are beyond the ability of one person to meet, even with some help.

It is rare to have a person with dementia cared for at home the whole time until they die from the disease causing their dementia. This is especially the case if they have no other major illness, as is often true for people who develop dementia under the age of sixty-five, which is called an 'early onset.' If, on the other hand, someone has another major chronic illness such as a heart condition, they may pass away from that condition before their dementia causes them to reach the final stage of brain deterioration.

Many times I heard a myth that "you can't die from dementia." This is not true. For the person who has only dementia, they eventually die because their brain is no longer able to keep them breathing, and their heart stops beating. They may also have developed pneumonia as one of the complications of lack of mobility, which has been caused by the dementia. In one instance where the person with dementia was in his fifties when he was diagnosed and when he died, he had no other illness and was quite fit. In the last stage before he died at home, there were two family carers who were fully dedicated to his care and they had help for many hours every day from other family members, paid caregivers and volunteers in order to cope with his care. Most people do not have the personal or financial resources to manage to care for the person with dementia at home until they pass away.

A person with dementia has a constellation of inabilities and difficulties that combine to produce the unique pattern of the expression of their disease at any one point in time. Each new inability interacts with the others to produce new challenges for the person with the disease and those supporting them. Whenever the progression of the disease changes the person's abilities and behaviours, the person affected, and their family, need to find new ways to cope with their care and daily life events.

In the early stage, many people with dementia continue to live on their own. They may develop new procedures and stick closely to those procedures, perhaps developing a reputation of being inflexible. If they have some help, they can continue living alone longer. They need assistance to shop, to go to doctor's (and other) appointments and to navigate the health care system generally. The more complex the activity, the more likely they are to need help to do it. As time goes by, they may need help with cleaning, cooking and personal care. Once the person with dementia starts to have difficulty with geographic orientation, and becomes so forgetful that they do not remember to eat, their safety is greatly compromised and they will fail to thrive if they continue to live alone. A severe weight loss, demonstrated by clothes that are far too big, and very poor grooming, may indicate that the person living alone with dementia needs help.

In rare instances, it happens that both members of a couple develop dementia simultaneously. They need outside help earlier than they would if one of them remained well. Carers of people with dementia need to continuously adapt to changes in the abilities of their loved one. People with dementia have a great deal of difficulty adapting to change. If both members of a couple have dementia, neither one can adapt to the changes in the other. There is usually a lot of conflict between them as a result. There are also very serious safety issues in this type of situation. Family members of such couples become overwhelmed and need much support.

If the person with dementia is living with another person who can become their carer, they are able to stay in their home much longer. The carer needs to continuously assess their own ability, strength and stamina to evaluate whether they are able to continue being the only carer, or if they need help. Dementia is unpredictable and the situation can change rapidly. Everything may be going well, however the nature of the next deterioration of the person with dementia may mean that the carer needs to take on a new element of the care of the person with dementia. This may mean a change in their pattern of daily life. The carer will feel like they are in a crisis until they figure out new ways of coping. For example, if they have gone shopping together up until this point, but the person with dementia suddenly is no longer able to go out in the car or to the plaza, their carer needs to change how often and when they go out, how long they can stay away, and may need to have someone stay with the person with dementia to ensure their safety. Often the person with dementia is fine on their own for an hour or two. Many carers do their errands early in the morning if their loved one with dementia always sleeps until late morning. Carers come to the realization that someone else needs to keep the person with dementia company while they are out, if they come home and find them extremely upset, or if there is chaos because the activity they attempted was too difficult for them to manage alone.

When the carer begins to feel a sense of panic that they just can't continue, that is a good sign that they need help from someone else. The next step is to figure out what would be most helpful. If they want to get out to a club meeting on their own, having someone come during that time may help. If they have a lot of contact already with friends and family, hiring someone to help with the household cleaning or the yard work may be the best choice. Carers can ask themselves "What work can I give away to someone else?" Family or neighbours may be able to provide the extra help needed. It is important for the carer to get help, in order to prevent their own health from deteriorating. Carers tend to put their own needs last, but it is completely legitimate and necessary for them to take care of their own health and well-being. If there is a day program for people with dementia available, the person with dementia will benefit from the stimulation it provides, but the decision of whether or not to use the day program more often rests with the need of the carer for a regular break.

As the person's dementia progresses, their care needs take up more and more of the time and energy of the carer. It is not the physical care needs that are the most demanding, but keeping the person with dementia emotionally calm as their misunderstandings result in increasing anxiety, and the time the carer needs to spend in redirection and engagement escalates. Some families are able to have regular family meetings to talk about the needs of the person with dementia and the needs of the main carer. They are able to compare how they cope and help each other with suggestions and solutions. Having a family member with dementia causes a shift in the life of the family, and regularly working together to help each other share the care of their family member will give the family new strength.

Understanding what stage the person with dementia is in makes it easier to decide if it is advisable to move. If the person with dementia is relying on their procedural memory to remain active and useful in the house, moving will disrupt that. If they are past the point where they are able to help out around the house, that will not be as important. If the carer feels they would rather stay in their own home after they are eventually alone, understanding how long the person with dementia is likely to remain there will help them decide whether they can continue to manage care of their home as well as care for the person with dementia. Staging is also helpful for financial planning for the future.

At some point, it is very likely that the carer will not be able to continue to provide care at home and needs to look for a nursing home for their loved one with dementia. There is no 'right' or 'wrong' time to do this. Some carers are able to manage until later in the disease process, some not as long. It depends primarily on the needs of the person with dementia and the health and well-being of the carer. Often the need for a nursing home comes up suddenly when dementia is the cause. The carer may be doing very well, but the next small deterioration that the person with dementia has, results in them having needs that the carer just cannot meet. These deteriorations are unpredictable, so therefore, when dementia is the cause, the need for a nursing home is also unpredictable. It is a good idea for the carer to have an emergency plan in place for how they will cope, in case the care needs of the person with dementia are suddenly overwhelming, while they wait for a bed in a nursing home to become available.

Having a loved one go into a nursing home is likely the most emotionally difficult experience the carer will ever have. The grief is extreme, and it is accompanied by guilt and a sense by the carer that they have failed the person with dementia. Many people spend months crying and wondering if they made the right decision. At the same time, they know that they are unable to provide the care that the person with dementia needs. It is important for the carer to recognize that they can continue to provide company and care to the person with dementia, and advocate on their behalf, even after they move into the nursing home.

It is important for the carer to keep some interest or activity that they do entirely for their own benefit throughout the course of their loved one's disease. The care needs of the person with dementia are so demanding that when they are suddenly no longer present, the former carer can lose all sense of purpose and identity. When the person with dementia moves into a nursing home or dies, that one interest or activity can be the start of rebuilding daily life for the carer.

7. The Challenge of Dementia

There is little physical pain with dementia, however the emotional pain, for the person with dementia, their carers and their extended community is enormously significant. We hope, every day, to hear on the news that there has been a scientific breakthrough, so that those who have dementia will be cured and these diseases will be eliminated. We must continue to hope and to support that research. However, we must also support the people who are currently struggling day by day, to give them understanding and care in order to lighten their burden.

What we have to offer is our presence and support to the person with dementia and to their carers. Being present is having a feeling of solidarity. Solidarity would come about by seeing the person with dementia with empathy and concern: a feeling that "it could be me in their shoes" and, also an attitude of "we're all in the same lifeboat together, so let's make the best of the ride."

The grief of the carers was described by one woman as being similar to the way she would have felt at a funeral. She felt as though people should be sitting with her, holding her hand, giving their condolences, and bringing food. However, she was aware that others around her saw her as having an ordinary day, caring for her husband with dementia, who was actually in the early stage of his illness. Dwelling with the diseases that cause dementia, means experiencing waves of grief while you are trying to learn about the best way to cope, deal with the expectations of others, and carry on with your other responsibilities. There is a disconnection between the way carers are feeling and how everyone else assumes they are feeling. It is important for carers to find support in their grieving, to have people to talk to who will understand and support you, as you dwell with dementia.

It's not just the tragic events of life that need discussing in order to feel emotional support. I remember calling a recently widowed family member daily for a few weeks because I knew he needed support. One day, he told me proudly that he had found underwear on sale at Kmart. Then he was a little embarrassed. However, I thought to myself, "That's what it takes to not feel alone. It takes having someone in your life who is interested in the small events of your life." If your spouse has dementia, you may or may not find such a person to give you that type of emotional support. However, it will help you feel stronger if you understand why you are sad. Otherwise, you feel like you have lost control of yourself.

Carers may get into a routine and feel that they are on top of their loved one's needs, only to feel devastated that all their efforts have not prevented their loved one from getting worse. There is cumulative grief, mounting up over all the losses and difficult to resolve, as they are still reminded of it since they are dwelling with the cause of their grief every day. This grief leads to anger, frustration, resentment, a sense of failure and other severe emotions. If you are the carer, you may feel grievous outrage because the person with the disease is no longer able to help you to meet your needs. You may feel anger because you don't have time to meet your own needs since you're so busy watching out for them. You will be extremely upset when people who are in a position to help you do not do so. You may feel frustration because you find yourself in so many strange situations in which you feel you have a real loss of control. You may not be able to re-establish control immediately; the situation just has to run its course.

One woman told me that after she understood that she was feeling stress because her situation was out of control, somehow that knowledge, by itself, lowered her stress. Her husband's condition had deteriorated and his anxiety was now so high that he was not sleeping at all. Of course, that meant she was unable to sleep as well. When we talked, she admitted that she felt she was inadequate; that if she could just find the right thing to say or do, he would be able to relax enough to sleep. This increased her own anxiety. Once she stopped blaming herself, her anxiety decreased. She did whatever she could for him, but stopped trying to "fix" the situation. She was able to survive with brief naps over a period of many weeks, while his physician tried changing some of his medications. Eventually, their home situation became more stable, but she did start the process of finding him a long-term care home after that. She realized that the crisis she had been through had taken a toll on her health, and she felt that she would be putting herself at risk if she continued to care for her husband at home.

Sometimes, when a person with dementia experiences a deterioration in their condition, it is relatively easy for the carer to alter their care patterns slightly. Other deteriorations place the person and their family in crisis because a more major change in care is needed, perhaps including medications. Normally, physicians prefer to change one medication at a time. If they change more than one, they are uncertain which change caused the alteration in the condition of the person with dementia. Therefore, finding a solution in terms of medication can take weeks. The course of the disease process can involve many crises, and it is unpredictable when these will occur.

Finding people to talk to, especially others who are experiencing the same things, in a support group, or on a carer web site may help give you strength to carry on. It is important to keep trying to find that support. For example, the Alzheimer Society (Canada) or Association (U.S.) provides support to people who are coping with any disease causing dementia. The website of Alzheimer's Disease International lists Alzheimer associations all around the world. Most Alzheimer associations also offer support to families whose loved one has a related disease causing their dementia, such as Frontotemporal dementia, Parkinson's disease with dementia, Vascular Dementia or Lewy Body disease. Specialized groups are also available, but may not be in your area. If there is no organization specializing in dementia near you, you may want to encourage some other organization close to you to start a group of people with similar needs. Support groups are very helpful for people who are looking for understanding to bolster their spirits and to sustain them through difficult times.

You will feel extreme shock and sadness that your loved one with dementia can no longer remember your friends or family. You may also feel embarrassed and tend to withdraw from friendships. Because of the great emotional toll on both of you, it is better to tell friends about the illness, seek their understanding, and maintain a social life together as long as possible. If the person with dementia reaches a point where they refuse to socialize, it is good for you to maintain friendships on your own. You need the strength that comes from strong supportive friendships and relationships with others. This is particularly true since the person with the disease is not able to fill the role of your companion in the same way they did in the past. One lady, whose husband had recently been diagnosed, and who was in the early stage, said, "Even when my husband is sitting in the chair right beside me, I miss him."

Some carers experience symptoms of depression (for example, problems with sleeping, decreased appetite, increased feelings of irritability, feelings of hopelessness). A family physician may suggest medication, such as an antidepressant, for the carer. This medication does not change your situation but may help you to cope more effectively. It is best to avoid getting into a pattern of substance abuse (excessive alcohol intake, addictive prescribed medications, or street drugs) in order to cope. Being a carer requires a lot of thoughtfulness, creativity, patience and perseverance, and is easier with a clear head. If you are feeling totally overwhelmed, you may need to seek help for support, new ideas or respite (someone else taking over your caring for a few days while you rest). Some carers find ways to spend time on activities, which they find helpful to relieve their stress. For example, one woman arranged to pay a carer to come for three hours a month so she could attend the monthly meetings of her horticultural club. She thought she could adjust to missing her other activities, but not that one club. A fellow looked after his wife lovingly, but went to a lot of trouble to arrange help so he could continue his regular weekly dart games with his friends. Looking after your own stress levels and health is very important.

Some people despair when their loved one has dementia. A few carers said that they thought their spouse had dementia because they, the carers, were being punished by God. When dementia is in your family, it could be viewed instead as a divine gift to teach totally unselfish caring. Viewing the dementia as a punishment means that a potential carer is starting out with cxccss guilt and resentment at being unfairly encumbered by a burden they don't deserve. This will make it difficult for them to view the person with dementia in a positive light. Quite a few carers of people with dementia voiced concern that their place of worship did not provide as much support to families where a member was dying of a disease causing dementia, when compared to the support offered to families of those with some other terminal illnesses. The long course of the illness, and the stigma about people with mental health issues, may have contributed to this lack of support. However, I did see some indication that the awareness of religious organizations concerning dementia is slowly changing.

Many carers are extremely proud of the care they give to their loved one in their time of need. Learning about dementia and receiving assistance from others in the community helps to alleviate despair, because the carers begin to feel a sense of accomplishment. Now and then people reach such a point of desperation that they consider ending their lives rather than going on. One fellow had a very concrete suicide plan all worked out. Nothing he tried to do, to help his wife with dementia, was working. Once he learned how to understand his wife, felt more successful at helping her, he was receiving regular emotional support, and assistance from a paid carer, he was able to carry on, and began to enjoy life again. Carers emerge from their experience as very strong people who are pleased that they were able to provide the care that their loved one needed. Many people who participated in activities with other carers, such as education and support groups, expressed their relief at knowing they weren't the only ones who were going through the experience of caring for a person with dementia. Since many personal issues are discussed at these groups, the firm rule is that personal information is not divulged outside the group. Many close friendships develop, which carry on long after the people with dementia have passed away.

As a society, our cultural acceptance of people with mental impairment needs to improve in order to give better support to people with dementia and their carers. There is a stigma about dementia. People, who tell others that they have dementia, are sometimes met with embarrassed silence, or denial. Most of the people with dementia I have worked with have told me that people have said to them. "You don't have Alzheimer's!" Now, would we say the same thing to someone who told us that they had been diagnosed with cancer? No; we would say something like: "I'm so very sorry. How are you feeling?" For some reason, people generally want to deny that there is any dementing disease present. They may attempt to minimize the difficulties that it presents by saying, "Don't worry, we all get a little forgetful at times." The people with dementia need to be validated; the people they are talking to need to accept that the diseases causing dementia are serious, and not to be dismissed lightly. People with early stage dementia appear normal, and, in the main, act normally. We expect that people with dementia will not do anything that appears normal, so when they say something that portrays wisdom and knowledge or do something that requires skill, it does not fit our expectation of how a person with dementia should be. Sometimes, in order to help myself judge my own responses, I compare them to what I would have said to someone who has terminal cancer, in order to measure whether I am being appropriate. Our culture has a stigma about cognitive illness and it is important to think about whether we are reflecting that stigma ourselves.

I remember hearing about a woman with dementia who had lived in an apartment building for many years and had many friends there. Once she developed dementia, her neighbours chose to start excluding her from their gatherings, and approached her family member, saying "She shouldn't be here!" This lady felt alone and rejected, which she was. When people with dementia are deprived of contact because they are rejected or excluded or kept on the outside of cliques, they experience a sense of social inferiority, which adds unnecessary suffering to their lives. It is important to stay connected, to maintain relationships as long as possible, so that all can feel a sense of belonging and connectedness. In order to help our friends and family members with dementia, we need to be more accepting and understanding of how they see the world and how they behave.

It is important for those who are not carers, to realize that they need to talk directly to the people with dementia. Often the behaviour of people with dementia indicates that they are not used to being talked to directly. When they stand beside their carer, their head is down and they remain pulled back from the conversation emotionally and physically. However, if you talk to them directly in a friendly manner, even to lightly pass the time, their head comes up, their shoulders go back and a big smile comes on their face as they look you in the eyes and respond.

It is a situation that has a lot of complexity. Many people with dementia indicate that they want to be treated as though they have normal cognition. At the same time, we also need to learn how to give them support in communication and in all other facets of life. Simultaneously, we need to give support to the other carers and stay strong ourselves. It is important to conquer our own fear about doing or saying the wrong thing, or at having to deal with someone else's unpredictability or potentially embarrassing behaviour. We need to be confident enough in ourselves that we can cope with confusion and unusual thinking and behaviour patterns in someone else. We also need to realize that if we make a mistake, we can fix it and carry on.

There is no easy way to lose a loved one from our lives. If it is sudden, it feels as though your whole world has changed in an instant, and your recovery can take years. If it is a prolonged illness, like dementia caused by a degenerative disease, the loss happens a little at a time and the grief builds over many years. Learning about the experience of the person with dementia helps their carers to understand their perspective and to design thoughtful dementia care. The carers can then be proud that they did their very best in caring for their loved one with dementia.

I'll leave the last word to a caring couple. After many years, this unusual fellow with dementia could still speak a little. In one of those heart-stopping moments of clarity, a few days before he died, he asked a question of his wife.

"Has this broken the family apart?"

"No," she replied, "It has brought us closer together."

"Oh, good."

Suggested Reading, References and Resources

Advocacy Centre for the Elderly. http://www.advocacycentreelderly.org/

Alzheimer's Disease International. http://www.alz.co.uk/finding-help

Alzheimer Society of Canada. http://www.alzheimer.ca/

Alzheimer's Society (UK). http://alzheimers.org.uk/

Alzheimer's Association (U.S.) http://www.alz.org/

Alzheimer Canada, Safely Home Wandering Registry. http://www.safelyhome.ca/

*Alzheimer's Store, The: An Ageless Design Company. http://alzstore.com/

Bell, Virginia and Troxel, David (2011). The Best Friends™ Approach to Alzheimer's Care. Health Professions Press, Inc.

Boss, Pauline (1999) Ambiguous Loss. Harvard University Press.

Boss, Pauline (2011). Loving someone who has dementia: How to find hope while coping with stress and grief. Jossey-Bass.

Camp, Cameron and Brush, Jennifer (1998) A therapy technique for improving memory: Spaced retrieval. http://www.myersresearch.org/.

Capossela, C. and Warnock, S. (1995, 2004). Share the Care™. http://www.sharethecare.org/

* Care Link Advantage: Independent Living Solutions. http://www.carelinkadvantage.ca/

Clinical Dementia Rating Scale. Washington University School of Medicine in St. Louis. Knight Alzheimer Disease Research Centre. http://alzheimer.wustl.edu/cdr/downloadselectionpage.htm

Cotter, Valerie T. (2005). Restraint free care in older adults with dementia. Keio J Med 54(2):80-84, June 2005. http://www.kjm.keio.ac.jp/past/54/2/80.pdf

Creasey, Dr. Helen "The Brain and Behaviour", a video produced by the University of Sydney (Australia) Television Service for the Alzheimer's Disease and Related Disorders Society (ADARDS).

Dementia Advocacy and Support Network. A worldwide organization by and for people with dementia.http://www.dasninternational.org/

Dempsey, Marge and Baago, Sylvia (1998) Latent Grief: The unique and hidden grief of carers of loved ones with dementia. American Journal of

Alzheimer's Disease and Other Dementias. March/April 1998, Vol. 13, #2, 84-91. http://aja.sagepub.com/content/13/2/84.abstract

Doidge, Norman (2007). The Brain That Changes Itself, Penguin Books. http://www.normandoidge.com/.

Dr. Beers' Criteria for Medications to Avoid in the Elderly. http://seniorjournal.com/NEWS/Eldercare/5-01-06BeersCriteria03-Tb1.htm

Early Warning Signs, Alzheimer Society of Canada http://www.alzheimer.ca/en/About-dementia/Alzheimer-s-disease/Warning-signs-and-symptoms/10-warning-signs

*Eyez-On. Personal GPS locators. http://www.eyez-on.com/

Fazio, Sam (1999). Rethinking Alzheimer's Care. Health Professions Press, Inc. Baltimore, MD, USA

* Forgetful Not Forgotten, http://www.forgetfulnotforgotten.com/

Gentle Persuasive Approaches as developed at St. Peter's Hospital in Hamilton, Ontario, Canada. http://www.ageinc.ca/gpa.php

Ghent-Fuller, Jennifer. (2002). Understanding the Dementia Experience. http://www.alzheimercambridge.on.ca/Understanding the Dementia Experience.pdf

Ghent-Fuller, Jennifer (2012). Thoughtful Dementia Care™: Understanding the Dementia Experience. http://www.understanding-dementia-experience.com/

*Hartford Insurance, The; Dementia and Driving; http://hartfordauto.thehartford.com/Safe-Driving/Car-Safety/Older-Driver-Safety/Dementia-Activity/

James, Oliver (2009). Contented Dementia. Vermillion, UK

Kertesz, Andrew (2006). The Banana Lady and Other Stories of Curious Behaviour and Speech. Trafford Publishing.

Kitwood, Tom (1997). Dementia reconsidered: The person comes first. Open University Press, UK.

Kuhn, Daniel (2004). Alzheimer's Early Stages. Hunter House Publishers.

Kuhn, Daniel and Verity, Jane. (2008). The Art of Dementia Care. Thomson Delmar Learning.

Lewy Body Dementia Association. http://www.lbda.org/

McFarlane, J.A and Clements, Warren (1994). The Globe and Mail Style Book. Penguin Books.

McGowin, Diana Friel (1993) Living in the Labyrinth, Delacorte Press.

Ontario Network for the Prevention of Elder Abuse.
http://onpea.org/english/trainingtools/index.html

Post, Stephen (1995, 2000) The moral challenge of Alzheimer's disease.
John Hopkins University Press.

Reisberg, B., Franssen, E.H., Hasan, S.M., Monteiro, I., Boksay, I., Souren,
L.E., Kenowsky, S., Auer, S.R., Elahi, S., and Kluger, A. Retrogenesis:
Clinical, physiologic, and pathologic mechanisms in brain aging,
Alzheimer's's and other dementing processes. European Archives of
Psychiatry and Clinical Neurosciences, 1999; 249(S3): 111/28-111/36.
http://www.ncbi.nlm.nih.gov/pubmed/10654097

Sabat, Steven R. Implicit memory and people with Alzheimer's disease:
Implications for caregiving. American Journal of Alzheimer's Disease and
Other Dementias, Vol. 21, #1, p. 11-14. Jan/Feb 2006.
http://aja.sagepub.com/content/21/1/11.extract

* Search and Rescue Research, dbS Productions, https://www.dbs-
sar.com/index.htm

Search is an Emergency: Preplan manual for the search and rescue of
missing people with Alzheimer disease and related dementias. Alzheimer
Society of Canada (2004). http://www.alzheimer.ca/en/We-can-
help/Resources/~/media/Files/national/For-
HCP/hcp_brochure_search_emerg_e.ashx

Stones, M., Ghent-Fuller, J., Bell, M., Malott, O., Clyburn, L., Stones, L.,
and Kalopack, P. (1997) Alzheimer disease and aggression: a guide for
caregivers. Captus Press.

Taylor, Richard (2007). Alzheimer's from the Inside Out.
http://www.richardtaylorphd.com/

Zgola, Jitka M. (1999) Care that works: A relationship approach to persons
with dementia. John Hopkins University Press.

All web sites were checked and found to be accurate as of June 12, 2012.

* Please note: The author is not personally endorsing these companies, but
rather, listing them to illustrate the types of products which are
commercially available.

About the Author

Jennifer Ghent-Fuller worked as a nurse in Canada for over twenty-five years, the last eleven as an educator and support counsellor for people with dementia and their families and other carers. Jennifer has a Bachelor of Arts from Queen's University (Kingston, Ontario), a Bachelor of Science in Nursing from the University of British Columbia (Vancouver, British Columbia), and a Master of Science in Nursing from the University of Western Ontario (London, Ontario). Jennifer has also worked as a volunteer in the fields of literacy and elder abuse prevention. She is now retired.

Made in the USA
San Bernardino, CA
11 March 2018